Conquer Obesity

Your Step-By-Step Guide to Lasting Weight Loss with the Gastric Balloon

ALEX BRECHER AND NATALIE STEIN

Copyright

Legal Disclaimer

Foreword

I was pleased and honored when I was asked to write the forward to *Conquer Obesity: Your Step-By-Step Guide to Lasting Weight Loss with the Gastric Balloon.*

Obesity is a worldwide disease that poses a major threat to the health of mankind. It is at such a point that the World Health Organization has created the term "Globesity" to refer to this pandemic. Traditionally, obesity is treated with conservative measures such as behavior modification, including diet and exercise, and medications. When facing severe obesity, bariatric surgery might be indicated. However, there remains a huge gap in treatment for patients for whom a conservative approach is sufficient, but who do not qualify for obesity surgery. With the approval of the intragastric balloon by the FDA in 2015, America now has another valid option to battle obesity.

Given my fifteen years of experience with intragastric balloons worldwide and more than two thousand balloons implanted, I consider this book to be really remarkable. It addresses the most important topics related to intragastric balloons with a major goal – helping the patient. The language is clear and concise, covering all steps that a patient needs to know about, from "what it is" to a clear description of when it is needed, the procedure highlights, and pre- and post-implant aspects. Besides informing people considering a balloon, this book will prepare people interested in the procedures for what to expect in each phase.

The information is gradually provided so as not to overwhelm the reader with too much information, and to make it easy to return to a specific piece of information for refreshing the memory. Special attention is given to diet planning, an issue that can always be confusing, no matter how much one knows about the topic.

No more with this book!

It is targeted to patients, and it provides the information from a patient's perspective in such a simple way that it will make it difficult for a physician to explain it better.

Also, the book will definitely be useful to bariatric endoscopy practices that can have it as a guide to help promote full patient understanding of the procedure in a language the patient can effectively understand.

Manoel Galvao Neto, MD

Assistant Professor of Surgery, Florida International University, Miami, USA

Bariatric Endoscopy Service chairman, Gastro Obeso Center, 9th of July Hospital, and Mario Covas Hospital ABC Medical School, Sao Paulo, Brazil

Innovation award recipient from the American Society of Metabolic and Bariatric Surgery in 2016

Letter from the Authors

Dear Reader,

Congratulations on your decision to learn about the gastric balloon or to get it! You're about to find out more about this tool that can help you lose weight, and also about to discover the healthy habits that can keep you losing weight and keep it off for years to come.

That's a big deal! If you're looking into the gastric balloon system, you've already been fighting obesity for quite a while. You've tried diets, and haven't found a permanent solution. The balloon is designed to lend a hand as you jump-start your weight loss. For 3 or 6 or even 12 months, the balloon will be in your stomach, reminding you of what you should and shouldn't eat.

When you get the gastric balloon, your doctor should also provide you with complete support. The balloon is supposed to be used along with a diet and exercise program that teaches you healthy habits for life. Regular visits with a nutritionist can get you on the right path and help you learn strategies for making the right choices.

This book is NOT a substitute for a complete nutritional and medical support program under the guidance of your own medical care team.

Your healthcare team may include your primary care physician, the doctor who put in your gastric balloon, a nutritionist, and any other healthcare experts you work with. We assume you also are working closely with your doctor and supporting team during the process.

This book can accompany you through your gastric balloon journey and is designed to assist you with each of the steps you will encounter on the gastric balloon experience from beginning to end.

It is set up in chapters that progress from learning about the gastric balloon and considering it, to losing weight with it, to life after the balloon is removed. It starts by giving you information about the balloon, moves forward with you as you get ready for the procedure, then as you lose weight for months with the gastric balloon. It will remain a valuable asset once you have the balloon removed and work to maintain the new lifestyle you will have adopted.

As you progress, we offer ideas and knowledge you will need to help you make healthy decisions and to make daily living easier. You will find practical advice on food choices, restaurants, and handling cravings. Along the way, we provide an assortment of healthy meal plans to help you plan your diet throughout your journey.

Most chapters also have a challenge to give you a chance to test your skills and your new awareness of nutrition, tools you can use, and how to develop habits that can help you lose weight and improve your health.

We hope this book can play a small role in your healthy gastric balloon journey. To your satisfying and long-lasting weight loss success!

Sincerely,

Alex and Natalie

Contents

Chapter 1

Introduction to the Gastric Balloon

THE GASTRIC BALLOON is an inflatable balloon that goes into your stomach. Depending on the manufacturer, the balloon or balloons are inflated with a saline, or salt water, solution, or with air. The inflated balloon system takes up space in your stomach so there is less space available for food.

The smaller amount of space available for food helps you fill up faster so it is easier to eat less. Eating less can help you lose weight. The system may also slow down the emptying of food from your stomach, so you feel full for longer after your meal.

Types of Balloon Systems

A few different companies make their own versions of gastric balloons. They all work in the same way: They take up space in your stomach so there is less room for food, and they slow stomach emptying so you feel full for longer. Each system is temporary, and you have it in for only 3 to 12 months before it is removed.

ORBERA Managed Weight Loss System[1]

The U.S. Food and Drug Administration approved ORBERA[2] in August 2015 for use as a weight-loss system in the United States.

The ORBERA balloon system stays in the stomach for up to six months. Your doctor will fill the balloon with about 1.5 to 2.5 cups of saline, depending on your body type.

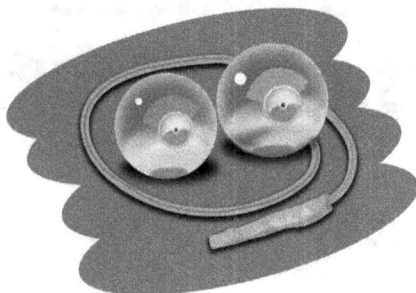

In one study cited by the FDA, patients lost an average of 10 percent of total body weight, or 22 pounds, by the end of the six months.

These patients maintained an average weight loss of 19 pounds by the end of nine months, or three months after balloon removal.

---

1   http://www.orbera.com/

2   http://www.fda.gov/MedicalDevices/ProductsandMedicalProce-
    dures/DeviceApprovalsandClearances/Recently-ApprovedDevices/
    ucm457416.htm

ReShape[3]

The FDA approved the ReShape Dual Balloon in July of 2015.[4] These balloons are filled with saline solution and also contain a dye called methylene blue that lets you know if there is a potentially dangerous leak.

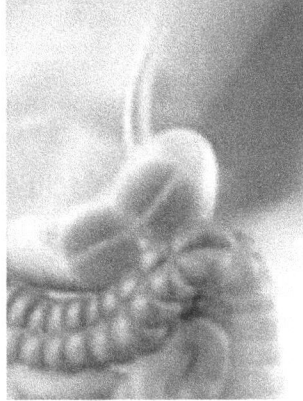

The ReShape Dual Balloon has a slightly different design than the ORBERA weight-loss system. ReShape Dual includes two interconnected balloons that stay in your stomach for six months.[5] The volume of each balloon is about 1.5 cups when filled with saline solution.

In an FDA clinical study, patients lost an average of 7.8 percent of total body weight, 9.9 pounds by the end of 48 weeks, or about six months after balloon removal.[6]

Spatz[7]

The Spatz Adjustable Balloon System is a single balloon. Unlike the ORBERA and ReShape systems, this balloon can stay

3   http://reshapeready.com/

4   http://www.fda.gov/MedicalDevices/ProductsandMedicalProcedures/DeviceApprovalsandClearances/Recently-ApprovedDevices/ucm456293.htm

5   https://reshapeready.com/about-reshape-non-surgical-weight-loss-procedure/

6   http://reshapeready.com/wp-content/uploads/2015/07/ReShape_Instructions_For_Use.pdf

7   http://reshapeready.com/

in your stomach for up to 12 months. A longer time in your stomach could possibly lead to more weight loss, and it gives you longer to develop new healthy lifestyle habits.

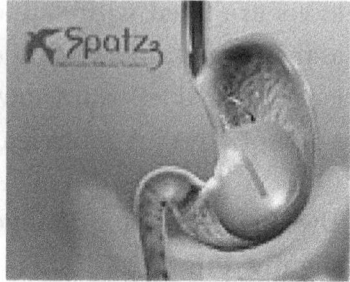

Another difference from the other balloon systems is that the Spatz balloon is adjustable. Your doctor can fill it more for greater inflation, or remove some of the saline solution to slightly deflate the balloon while it is in your stomach. You may need the balloon inflated further if you need more restriction to help you lose weight. Deflation can be necessary if the balloon is too uncomfortable or is not letting you eat enough.

As of March of 2016, the Spatz Adjustable Balloon System was not FDA-approved in the United States. The system has been approved as an obesity treatment in Canada and countries in Europe, the Middle East, South America, Asia, and Africa.

Obalon[8]

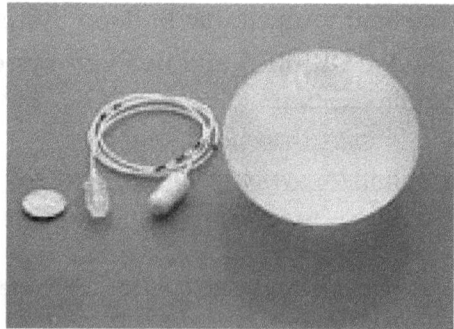

The Obalon balloon is another balloon system that works similarly to the others but is filled with air instead of saline. You can have a single small balloon or two, or even three Obalon balloons. Each balloon can be filled to about 1 cup.

8   http://www.obalon.com/

The Obalon balloon is typically used for only 12 weeks, which is less than you're likely to have the balloons made by the other companies.

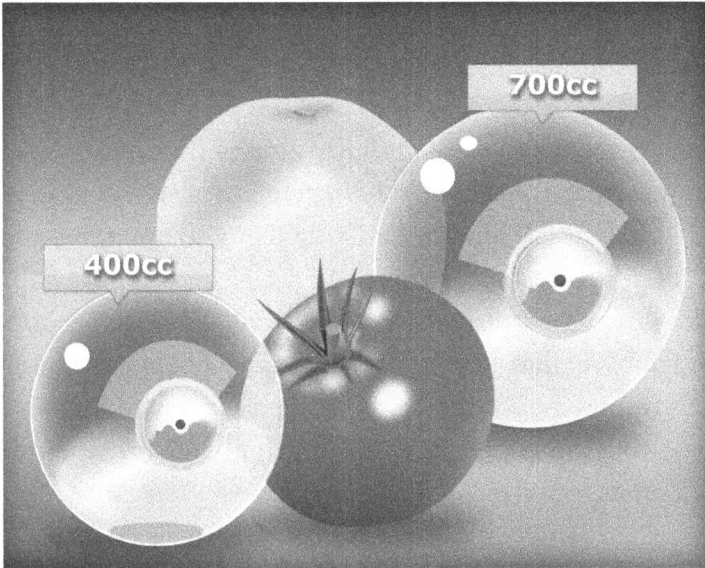

A 700cc balloon is about the size of a grapefruit. A 400cc balloon is about as big as a tomato.

Balloon Placement and Removal

The Basic Steps

Once you look into the gastric balloon and decide that it's for you, you can start planning your weight-loss journey. You can work with your doctor and healthcare team to schedule your procedure and to set short-term and long-term weight loss goals. You can also talk about strategies for losing weight and keeping it off after the balloon is removed.

Nausea and vomiting are common in the first few days after you get the balloon. You will need to be on a liquid diet to reduce discomfort as you adjust to the balloon. Your doctor may also prescribe medications that will make the symptoms more manageable. Most patients can return to work and regular activities within days.

For the three to six months that you have the balloon system in your stomach, you should follow a controlled diet under the supervision of your doctor, nutritionist, and any other members of your healthcare team. The goal here is to establish healthy eating patterns that can last you for life. Adopting a regimen of regular exercise also can also help in weight loss, weight maintenance, and general health. You can expect to lose 15 to 25 or more pounds with the balloon if you follow your diet as recommended.

After the balloon comes out, your job will be to continue the healthy lifestyle patterns you practiced while you had the balloon. This can help you continue to lose weight and to keep the weight off. If possible, you can follow up with your doctor and nutritionist to stay on track and keep learning.

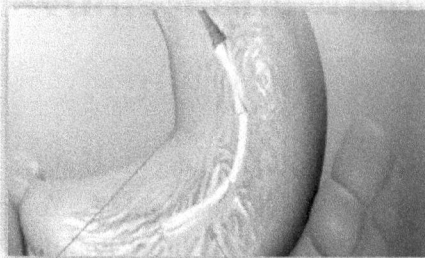

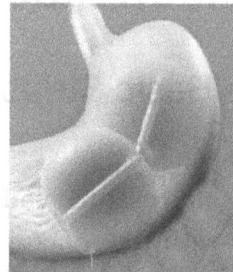

At left, the balloon system is inserted by catheter into the stomach, then inflated, at right, or filled with saline solution.

Getting the Balloon

Balloon placement and inflation is an outpatient procedure that typically takes less than 30 minutes. You will be asked not to eat or drink anything for 12 hours before your appointment to prevent the risk of choking while you are under sedation. Ask your doctor about whether you should continue to take any medications that you are on.

You will receive a mild sedative. The doctor places the balloon or balloons in your stomach and then fills it with a saline solution. When full, a single balloon may contain about 1.5 to 2.5 cups of solution and is about the size of an orange or grapefruit.

When filling the balloon, the doctor may also place a blue dye in your balloon. If the balloon breaks, dye will leak out and you will see it in your urine. If you do, you need to call your doctor immediately.

Also call your doctor if you notice pain or redness in your arm where the IV was placed for the anesthesia. Also, let your doctor know if you do not urinate within 12 hours of leaving the doctor's office. You may be dehydrated.

You may have some pain after the procedure. Your doctor can prescribe pain medication if necessary. Plan to take it easy the day of the procedure. You cannot drive after getting anesthesia, and you should not make important decisions since you may be a little groggy.

The procedure for getting the Obalon balloon is a little different. You swallow a capsule that contains the balloon. Then the doctor inflates the balloon through a tube, and then removes the tube. The doctor can then add another balloon or two. The whole procedure can take about 15 minutes, and you don't need sedation.

Balloon Use and Removal

The length of time the balloon remains in your stomach depends on the brand of the balloon and on your doctor's recommendations. You need to get the balloon out as recommended, because keeping it in longer can be dangerous. The balloon can deflate and cause a bowel obstruction.

During the time the balloon is in your stomach, you should work with your healthcare team to follow a healthy, reduced-calorie diet that can help you lose weight. When the balloon comes out, your job will be to maintain your weight loss and healthier lifestyle. You can do this by continuing to follow the healthy diet you were developed when you had the balloon in your stomach.

Is the Balloon for You?

The gastric balloon is for patients who have a BMI (body mass index) of 30 to 40 kg/m^2. That's 175 to 233 pounds for a 5'4" woman, or 209 to 278 pounds for a 5'10" man. Your doctor may recommend the balloon if you have been unsuccessful at permanently losing weight using conventional diet and exercise programs, and if you have one or more health problems related to extra weight.

You should also be ready to commit to an intensive diet and lifestyle program while you have the balloon, and be ready to continue these changes after the balloon comes out.

Who Shouldn't Get the Balloon?

The balloon is not for you if:

- You have a serotonin syndrome; this is a greater concern for ReShape and you may be able to get a different balloon.

- You take prescription gastric irritants such as aspirin or anticoagulants.

- You have liver problems.

- You are pregnant or breastfeeding.

- You have had weight-loss surgery or any gastric surgery.

How Much Weight Will You Lose?

The amount of weight you lose depends on the exact diet you follow, the amount of exercise you do, and your weight. Many patients lose 25 percent to 50 percent of their excess body weight, or about 15 percent of total body weight.

In one study, patients with the balloon lost an average of 21 pounds at the end of six months, compared with an average of 7 pounds among patients without the balloon who just received diet and exercise counseling. The balloon was removed after six months. By one year, the patients who had used the balloon had an average weight loss of 16 pounds.

Gastric Balloon Safety

The gastric balloon is far less invasive than weight loss surgery, but there are some possible risks. In clinical trials of the leading gastric balloons, these were some of the more serious side effects that were reported.

- Vomiting

- Stomach or abdominal pain

- Esophageal puncture or damage

- Pneumonia

- Dehydration

There also is a chance that you could have intolerance to the balloon system and need it taken out, especially within the first 2-3 weeks.

Additional side effects that are relatively common, but not considered serious are:

- Indigestion

- Ulcers

- Heartburn

- Constipation and/or diarrhea

- Decreased appetite

- Dizziness

Practitioner requirements

To be able to offer the gastric balloon and related weight loss program, your doctor should:[9]

- Be skillful in advanced upper endoscopy and inter-ventional endoscopy.

- Complete a training program to be able to offer the balloon.

- Use the balloon as part of comprehensive weight loss program that includes long-term support and follow up.

- Include multidisciplinary support from specialists such as a nutritionist, psychologist, radiologist, and exercise counselor or physical therapist.

- Provide relevant training for support staff.

Maintaining Weight Loss

To maintain weight loss, it is up to you to continue to follow the healthy, portion-controlled diet and good eating habits you learned and practiced when you had the balloon system in your stomach. Continuing a regular exercise program also is highly recommended.

Each of the following chapters has some suggested daily menus or meal plans to help you lose weight. Assuming your doctor and nutritionist approve, you can follow the meal plans exactly, or you can modify them to meet your needs.

---

9   http://www.orbera.com/resource/1450978093000/o_orbera_code/pdf/
     ORBERA_Directions_for_Use_GRF-00346-00R01.pdf

For example, you can always substitute foods from a similar food group. Appendix A has lists of healthy foods and their food groups and serving sizes. Here are some sample substitutions:

- **Swap a serving of protein for a serving of another protein.** If the meal plan says 3 ounces of chicken, you can have 3 ounces of tuna, ½ cup of non-fat cottage cheese or tofu, 1 egg, or any other single serving of protein you like.

- **Swap a serving of vegetables for a serving of other vegetables.** If the meal plan says 1 cup of steamed broccoli, you can have a cup of cauliflower, zucchini, carrots, or any other cooked or raw non-starchy vegetable, or 2 cups of salad greens. And you can always have more vegetables than the plan calls for!

- **Swap a starch for another starch.** If the meal plan calls for 2 slices of whole-wheat bread, you can have 1 cup of high-fiber cereal, ½ cup cooked whole grain pasta or brown rice, a small sweet potato, or any other high-fiber, nutritious starch.

- **Swap a fruit for a fruit.** If your menu says 1 medium apple, you could have a medium orange or pear, or 1 cup of berries, grapes, or cut melon, or any other serving of fruit.

You can also make the meal plan your own by dividing up the meals and snacks however you prefer. You can have the number of meals and snacks that works best for you. Some people like three bigger meals, while others prefer three smaller meals and three snacks, while others are somewhere in the middle.

THE CHALLENGES

The following chapters each have a challenge for you to do. Don't worry – they're not graded! They're just a chance for you to practice what you learned, or to develop new healthy habits that will take you far as you lose weight and beyond.

Each challenge is simple, and you can get started with the guidelines that are there.

Chapter 2

Getting Ready for the Balloon

Managing Your Weight: New Hope with the Balloon

WHY ARE YOU getting the gastric balloon? Why do you think it will help you when other diets have not worked for you? What will you do to make sure you are successful with the balloon? We'll look at these questions as you prepare to get your balloon.

If you're considering the gastric balloon chances are that diets have not worked for you. You may have been able to lose a few pounds or a lot of weight when you followed a diet, but the weight came back after stopping the diet. Often, the weight – plus a few extra pounds – came back!

The hope with the gastric balloon is that it will not only help you lose weight, but keep it off. During the months you have the balloon, you will be learning about nutrition and practicing healthy eating strategies that you can keep up for the long-term. It's not so much about going on a diet as adopting a new lifestyle.

A Long-Term Solution

The gastric balloon is designed to help you lose weight as you develop the healthy eating habits that will last for life. As you progress through the program, you can learn more about healthy eating choices and strategies for staying true to them and to yourself. This guide is designed to help you move forward so that by the time you get rid of the balloon system, you are confident you can and will keep the weight off.

To be as successful as possible with the gastric balloon, you need to take a long, hard look at your lifestyle and be brutally honest with yourself. What has gone wrong in the past? Why are you struggling with your weight now? Is it because you eat mindlessly? Are you a victim of emotional eating who turns to food for comfort, celebration, and companionship? Are you a boredom eater? Do you eat too fast? Do you choose high-calorie foods?

Once you identify what your challenges have been, you can work to address them. If you are a boredom eater, for example, you can make a list of non-eating activities to do instead of eating when you are bored. Emotional eaters can try to get to the root of the problem, and also come up with strategies such as phoning a friend or taking a walk when their feelings get overwhelming. We will help guide you through this process in later chapters.

You're not in this Alone

As you work through your journey with the gastric balloon, you will need to remember that this is NOT a solo venture. You have many changes in your lifestyle to undertake and you will need the help and understanding not only of your healthcare team, but also of those closest to you and, perhaps, of people who you have yet to meet.

It will be helpful for you to consider those closest to you as you work to understand why previous weight-loss efforts have not resulted in lasting change, and enlist them in your renewed efforts to use the gastric balloon to succeed in your journey to a healthier weight and lifestyle.

And as you seek to learn more about nutrition, healthy food choices, exercise and all the pros and cons of the many choices you may consider, you will find yourself reaching out to new people and organizations who can provide lasting resources and support.

Health and Family: A Perfect Pairing

As you develop your healthy habits as part of your gastric balloon journey, they will become part of your regular life. You may find it beneficial to incorporate your family into your new regimens, both to encourage change that involves them and also as support.

For example, you may want to include your children and spouse as much as possible in all parts of your food preparation from grocery shopping to cooking. They can help you read labels and find healthy choices at the store, or discover new healthy recipes in books or on the internet. You can even play games such as thinking of fun ways to cook healthy ingredients such as eggplants or tofu.

The same is true for activity. As you develop an exercise program, it may become something you usually do on your own early in the morning or late in the evening, but it's also something that can be part of family life. You can help your children practice sports, or plan family outings that involve fun exercise. You can rent bikes, go swimming or hiking, walk around a fun downtown area, or take balls and other sports equipment for a fun day at the park.

It doesn't need to take much time or be fancy. The little things you do add up to calories burned for you, and set a good example for the rest of your family. Some simple, everyday examples include:

- Walking your children to or from school. This is a great opportunity for family time, too.

- Taking an after-dinner walk with your spouse and/ or children.

- Parking in a single spot and walking to several nearby stores to get errands done. For example, you could park at the grocery store so you do not have to carry heavy bags, and walk to the library, post office, or any other places within range to finish your errands.

- Making it a habit to park in a far spot in the parking lot or even a few blocks away.

The active time you spend together builds bonds, creates memories, helps your family build their own healthy habits, and burns extra calories.

Support from All Sides

As you prepare for the balloon, you also should begin to build up your support system for when you need some encouragement or extra motivation. You can think of your support system as holding you up in the center. If you have support all around you, you can't fall down. You can only lean so far before your support catches you and helps to prop you back up and keep you on track.

Your significant other, close relatives, and friends are ideal candidates. They already support you in the rest of your life when you have issues at work and in other parts of your life. They might as well help you through this, too.

They can help by simply listening when you have a rough day of eating or a disappointing weigh-in. They can go further by walking with you and agreeing not to eat too much junk food with you. If you want, you can even ask them to help keep you on track by asking you how your weight loss is going, or by mentioning if you seem to be eating too many unhealthy foods.

If you have children, they can also be part of your support system. Just make sure not to burden them with your troubles. Instead, it may be more appropriate for your children to support you without realizing it.

Let children cheer you up by making sure to be grateful for them and show them you love them. And, let them motivate you as you think about being as healthy as possible for them. You want to be around for a lot of years, and you want to be active and healthy for those years!

Even your colleagues can be part of your system. They're especially helpful because you spend so much time at work, and work can be an especially unhealthy place if it is filled with breakroom doughnuts and other goodies. In your honest assessment of previous efforts at dieting and weight control, you probably will have identified areas here you may need their help to conquer.

If you have one or more colleagues that you're friendly with, talk to them about your plans and ask them to help you out, the same way your friends and family help you out at home. You may be a little shy, but you can also ask coworkers who are trying to lose weight for help. You'd be surprised at how much they might appreciate someone like you who can support them at work as you both try to pack healthy lunches and take walks at lunch.

Build Your Possible Resources – More Help

Going it alone is the tough way to go, so don't even try it! You have plenty of options for getting answers and inspiration whenever you need it. These are some go-to resources that can get you where you need to go.

A weight loss buddy can be your most valuable resource. You two can cheer on each other's triumphs, and sympathize with the challenges that the weight loss journey brings. You can hold each other accountable to exercising and eating right.

You may not be able to find a gastric balloon buddy, but that's okay. Anyone wanting to lose weight is going through similar challenges in eating right and staying on track. A non-balloon buddy can learn a bit about your unique challenges, and may even be able to offer some useful suggestions from an outside perspective.

Discussion forums can also be helpful. They're available 24/7, so you can expect answers at all hours of the day and night, which may be when you have your biggest crises! They're also great because you are unlikely to meet the other members in person and you can post anonymously if you want. That can give you the courage to post things you might otherwise feel are too embarrassing. In addition, forums give you the chance to post at any time that is convenient for you, and others can respond when they log on sooner or later.

The internet has plenty of good information about the gastric balloon and healthy eating. Usually, information provided by universities, the government, and established hospitals and healthcare systems is trustworthy and accurate.

Still, there is a lot of misinformation online, too! Special interest groups may have their own agendas and post information that is misleading. It's a red flag if you're asked to purchase something!

People who are misinformed may post information that is flat-out wrong. Remember, anyone is allowed to post anything online. It is not necessarily true just because you saw it on a blog, forum, or on another site.

Picking out the good from the bad information can be a challenge. If you're not sure, ask your gastric balloon doctor, one of your regular doctors, or your nutritionist. They might also be able to suggest more websites to visit.

Getting a Head Start with Some Basic Nutrition

The core of the program is your diet, so it makes sense to have a bit of basic nutrition knowledge. You'll be using your nutrition expertise along the way while you have the balloon in place and while you keep losing weight during life after the balloon. A little bit of information will go a long way, so here goes!

Calories: Energy and Weight Control

Calories are at the foundation of weight control. A calorie is a unit of energy. Protein, carbohydrates, and fat in food are sources of energy, or calories. Food energy fuels your heartbeat, breathing, body temperature regulation, and muscle movements.

Sounds good, right? The problem is, too much of a good thing is bad.

Your body only needs so many calories. When you get too many calories from food, or you eat too much, the extra calories are stored as body fat. You gain weight, feel sluggish, and eventually you can have trouble with blood sugar control, high blood pressure, and high cholesterol.

The gastric balloon helps you eat less, so you take in fewer calories. When you burn more calories than you take in, you lose weight. Ideally, you can take in calories from healthy sources of protein, carbohydrates, and fats so you can satisfy hunger without gaining weight. The balloon helps with that.

If you're going to count one thing while losing weight, it should be calories. A good goal for most people to start with is 1,200 calories. That's low enough to lose weight, but high enough to stay nourished if you make healthy choices. Later, when you are maintaining your weight, you might be as high as 2,000 calories or more, especially if you are a taller man and are active.

Protein: Sustained Energy and Lean Muscle Mass

Protein gets a lot of attention, and for good reason. Protein is a nutrient your body uses to make muscles, bones, and other tissues like skin and hair. You also need protein for a strong immune system, healthy metabolism, and normal hormone function.

Protein is also a good nutrient for weight loss because it helps you feel full. Protein slows down the emptying of food from your stomach after you eat, so you feel full for longer after a meal. That can help you eat less at the next meal.

How much protein should you get? Your body can only use so much protein for protein-related functions. That is, more protein doesn't lead to more energy, more lean muscle mass, and more weight loss. Protein has 4 calories per gram, and eating more than you need leads to fat storage and weight gain. Over time, very high levels of protein can even cause liver and kidney damage.

So, a good goal is about 75 to 120 grams of protein per day. That's 25 percent to 40 percent of your calories on a 1,200-calorie diet, or 15 percent to 24 percent of calories in a 2,000-calorie diet. That's right within the range for a long-term, sustainable diet plan.

The best sources of protein are nutrient-dense, lean foods. Here are some proteins to choose and to limit.

Choose These	Limit These
Fish and shellfish	Fatty meats and chicken and turkey with skin: they are high in calories and in artery-clogging saturated fat.
Beans, lentils, and split peas	Most deli meats: they can contain nitrates, which cause cancer, and usually also are high-sodium.
Soybeans, tofu, soy burgers, and other soy-based products	Fatty processed meats: they're high in calories, artery-clogging saturated fat, sodium, and nitrates.
Reduced-fat dairy products: yogurt, cheese, cottage cheese, and milk	Full-fat dairy products: they have unnecessary extra calories.
Skinless chicken and turkey	Protein shakes: they can be high in sugar and artificial ingredients. Even if not, they're liquid forms of calories and not as satisfying as real food.
Lean beef	
Lean ground beef, chicken, and turkey	
Eggs and egg whites	
All-natural, low-sodium deli meats such as turkey breast and lean ham	
Nuts, seeds, and peanuts	

You can also check Appendix A for a list of healthy proteins to choose.

Carbs: The Secret to Energy and Fat-Burning Secret

Carbohydrates have quite the mixed reputation. Recently, they have been blamed for everything from weight gain, to food cravings, to diabetes and more. Carbohydrates provide 4 calories per gram, and they are your body's main source of energy.

Not all carbohydrates and foods with carbohydrates are the same when it comes to health and your weight. Some carbs, like simple sugars (think of candy, baked goods, and soda) and refined starches (think of white bread, white rice, and white pasta) drive up your blood sugar levels and can make you hungrier within an hour or so when the spike recedes.

Other, high-fiber carbs (think of beans, winter squash, and unsweetened shredded wheat) are more satisfying. They digest more slowly and help keep your blood sugar and energy levels stable for hours.

How many carbs should you have per day? A good goal is about 150 grams if you are on a 1,200-calorie diet. That's about 50 percent of your daily calories. If you are hitting about 2,000 calories overall, your goal might be closer to 300 grams a day, or 60 percent of your total calories.

That number may be higher than a low-carb dieter's goal, but it may be a more sustainable goal for the long-term. With at least 150 grams of carbs a day, you have plenty of room for healthy choices like oatmeal, beans, and sweet potatoes, and even a little space for the occasional planned treat.

Choose These	Limit These
Whole grain breads	Sugar-sweetened drinks: they don't add nutrition, and they pile on the sugar and calories.
Whole grain pasta, brown rice, barley, and other whole grains	Desserts, such as cakes, pies, cookies, and muffins: they're high in calories, sugar, and refined grains, plus they often are high in unhealthy fats without adding essential nutrients.
Oatmeal and other hot and cold whole grain cereals	White breads, bagels, pita, English muffins, and other breads: they're refined grains that can spike blood sugar.
Fresh and frozen fruit	White rice, white pasta, refined cereal, and other refined grains: they can spike blood sugar.
Beans, split peas, and lentils	Fruit juice and dried fruit: they're calorie-dense, high in sugar, and not too filling.
Sweet potatoes, winter squash, and other starchy vegetables	
Non-starchy vegetables	
Reduced-fat dairy product	

Fat: Calorie Bombshell, but Necessary for Weight Loss

Fat can easily lead to weight gain. It has 9 calories per gram – more than twice the calories as a gram of carbohydrates or protein! Plus, your body can digest and store it very easily. Eat too much fat, and you'll definitely see the results on your belly, hips, and wherever else you tend to store fat.

On the other hand, like carbohydrates, fats are necessary for weight loss and health. Fat is slow to digest and keeps you satisfied for longer after a meal. It also helps keep blood sugar levels from spiking like they do when you eat a bunch of carbs.

You may have heard about good fats and bad fats. The bad ones are trans fats and saturated fats, which your body does not need. They generally increase your risk for heart disease and can even lead to diabetes and other chronic conditions. Plus, they're often contained in unhealthy, high-calorie foods – think fried foods, ice cream, and bacon.

The "good" fats are the ones to focus on. They can help you lose weight if you consume them in moderate amounts. They also lower your risk for heart disease. The best ones are monounsaturated fats, such as are found in avocados, peanuts, nuts, and olive oil, and Omega-3 fats, such as are found in fish, walnuts, and flaxseed.

Choose These (Small Serving Sizes)	Limit These
Avocados	Butter: it can be high in saturated fat.
Oli ve oil	Lard: it can be high in saturated fat.
Canola oil	Shortening: it can be high in trans-fat.
Other vegetable oils	Foods with "partially hydrogenated oil" as an ingredient: they can be high in trans-fat.
Nuts and peanuts	Fatty meats and cheeses: their fat is mainly saturated.
Sunflower, pumpkin, and other seeds	
Flaxseed	
Fatty fish	

So, how much fat should you get? A good goal is about 30 grams in a 1,200-calorie diet, which is about 23 percent of calories. You can shoot for about 40 to 70 grams on a 2,000-calorie diet, or about 18 to 31 percent of calories from fat.

The Other Nutrients – Stay Healthy and Feel Great

Vitamins and minerals are not directly related to weight loss since they do not contain calories. However, they're essential for health, healthy metabolism, and energy. The best way to hit your vitamin and mineral requirements is to eat a varied diet full of nutritious foods – think unprocessed, whole foods rather than processed foods.

If you eat a balanced diet with a variety of healthy foods, there's a good chance you will meet your nutrient requirements from food alone. That's not necessarily the case for everyone, though. You might fall short when you're cutting your calories to lose weight. You can also fall short if you avoid certain food groups, or if for some reason your body needs additional nutrients.

If you think you may be falling short of necessary nutrients, you can consider adding supplements. Taking supplements does not mean you have failed at designing a healthy diet; it could just mean you are looking for an insurance policy against nutritional deficiencies.

Nutrients of Concern

Your body needs more than 30 vitamins, minerals, and other nutrients to survive. Many of them are not of concern because they're in lots of foods or you don't need very much of them.

Others are more worrisome because they're not in very many foods, or you need more of them.

These are some of the nutrients of concern and the foods that are their best sources. You might consider taking supplements if you do not regularly eat these foods.

- **Calcium:** Milk, cheese, yogurt, fortified soy, almond, and cashew milk, canned bony fish like sardines, some fortified breakfast cereal.

- **Iron:** Meat, poultry, seafood, beans, nuts, fortified grains, leafy green vegetables.

- **Vitamin B12:** Seafood, meat, poultry, milk, yogurt, cheese, eggs.

- **Vitamin D**: Fortified milk, fatty fish such as salmon, eggs.

- **Omega-3 fatty acids:** Seafood, walnuts, flaxseed and flax oil, chia seeds.

Do talk to your doctor or nutritionist before taking any supplements. Some can be dangerous if you take too much of them or take them when you do not need them. Calcium, for example, is necessary for bone health, but too much can lead to heart trouble. Before you start taking supplements, and within a few months after you start, your doctor should measure your levels of various nutrients.

You can also take a multivitamin and mineral supplement to meet your needs, and talk to your doctor about particular concerns. These are some of the most common ones:

- Calcium and vitamin D for strong bones.

- Iron to prevent anemia and fatigue, especially in women.

- Vitamin B12, especially if you are an older adult or eat a plant-based, vegan diet.

YOUR CHALLENGE

Your challenge for now is to get your kitchen ready for weight loss. Before you get the balloon is a good time to clean out your kitchen and stock it up with healthy foods.

Out with the Bad

If you have any problem foods, getting rid of them now will keep them from tempting you later. You might want to get rid of any foods you know are triggers for overeating. They could be ice cream, brownie mixes, fatty meats like bacon and sausage, fatty cheese, and snack foods such as cookies, chips, dip, and crackers.

In with the Good

At the same time, you can stock up on some staples. When you have a well-stocked kitchen, you can make healthy meals. You're less likely to opt for take-out or delivery when an easy meal is close at hand. These are some staples to consider keeping in your pantry and freezer.

In your pantry:

- Canned tomatoes and tomato sauce.

- A full range of dried herbs and spices.

- Unsweetened almond milk.

- Canned tuna and any other kind of canned sea-food you like, such as salmon, sardines, oysters, and clams.

- Olive oil.

- Oatmeal and whole-grain cereal.

- Brown rice, whole-grain pasta, and other whole grains such as barley.

- Dried or low-sodium canned beans, split peas, and lentils.

- All-natural peanut butter.

- Vinegar.

- Condiments such as yellow and deli mustard and low-sodium soy sauce.

- Snacks such as brown rice cakes and plain popcorn.

In your freezer:

- Frozen fruit such as blueberries, strawberries, peaches, and any of your other favorites (check to make sure they have no added sugar).

- Frozen vegetables such as spinach, broccoli, cauli-flower, green beans, and mixed vegetables such as stir fry blends (check to make sure the veggies have no added salt).

- Frozen lean proteins such as chicken breasts, veggie burgers, fish fillets (not breaded), and ground turkey patties.

- Frozen whole-grain English muffins and waffles or pancakes.

You can get your fresh produce and perishable refrigerator items after you get the balloon and are ready to start eating solid foods. These types of items can include:

- Yogurt and other dairy products, such as non-fat cottage cheese and low-fat or nonfat cheese, such as string cheese, feta, and cheddar.

- Eggs.

- Salad greens, such as lettuce, spinach, baby greens, arugula, and bagged salad mixes.

- Salad vegetables, such as tomatoes, cucumbers, radishes, and mushrooms.

- Vegetables for snacking or cooking, such as cabbage, eggplant, bell peppers, broccoli, onions, and Brussels sprouts.

- Fruit such as apples, oranges, berries, and melon.

- Quick proteins such as tofu, cooked chicken breast, and all-natural deli meat.

Making the Kitchen Chef-Ready

Let's face it. When your kitchen counters are covered with clutter and you can't find your chef's knife, vegetable peeler, mixing bowls, and baking pans, it's easier to hit your smartphone up for pizza delivery than it is to cook a healthy meal.

Clean and organize your kitchen so it's a welcoming place to cook. Clear the papers and schoolbooks from your counters. Organize your kitchen drawers so you know where the cutlery, pots, and utensils are. Get yourself a set of containers with tight-fitting lids so you can store your food easily.

Set aside a few hours or days to get your kitchen ready for weight loss. It will be one of the most helpful steps you take before getting the balloon.

THE MEAL PLAN

Now you've decided to get the balloon, you've thought about how you're going to make the balloon system work for you in the short term and long term, and you know a bit about the basic nutrients. It's time to schedule your procedure!

As you look forward to it, you can follow a basic, balanced diet to get your body ready to lose weight. Here's a sample day. It has about 1,400 calories. That may be more than what you will have with the gastric balloon, but it is probably less than you have been eating, and it can help you lose weight.

Meal 1

Meal	Menu
Breakfast	1 cup Cheerios ½ cup skim milk ½ banana, sliced ½ ounce sliced toasted almonds
Lunch	Turkey sandwich: ✓ 2 slices of whole wheat bread ✓ 2 slices (1 ounce) all-natural turkey breast ✓ 1 slice low-fat cheese ✓ (Optional) deli, Dijon, or yellow mustard ✓ (Optional) Lettuce, tomatoes, sprouts, and/or onions 1 cup cherry or grape tomatoes 1 medium pear or apple
Snack	1 cup fat-free Greek yogurt

Meal	Menu
Dinner	Chicken with artichokes: ✓ One 4-ounce chicken breast stewed with 2 teaspoons olive oil, ✓ ½ 15-ounce can of artichoke hearts ✓ 1 cup fresh spinach leaves ✓ capers ✓ lemon juice ✓ pepper to taste ½ cup cooked brown rice mixed with 2 ounces of avocado

Meal 2

Meal	Menu
Breakfast	Breakfast sandwich: ✓ 1 whole-grain English muffin ✓ 2 tablespoons peanut or almond butter ✓ 1 medium apple, sliced ✓ Cinnamon, optional
Lunch	Tuna egg salad: ✓ ½ cup canned tuna ✓ ¼ cup fat-free sour cream or Greek yogurt ✓ 1 hard-boiled egg ✓ ½ cup cooked chopped cauliflower ✓ Pepper, Dijon mustard, and onion and garlic powder to taste ½ cup non-fat cottage cheese with 2 tablespoons sunflower seeds
Snack	1 cup baby carrots ¼ cup hummus

Meal	Menu
Dinner	Spaghetti and meatballs: ✓ ½ cup whole grain spaghetti ✓ ½ cup low-sugar, low-fat marinara or tomato sauce Meatballs made with: ✓ 3 ounces of lean ground turkey or soy crumbles ✓ Italian seasoning ✓ garlic powder ✓ black pepper 1 cup cooked vegetables, such as broccoli and carrots Side salad with 2 cups lettuce, fresh tomatoes and cucumbers 2 tablespoons vinaigrette (or 2 teaspoons olive oil and 1 tablespoon red wine or balsamic vinegar)

Chapter 3

Living with the Balloon

CONGRATULATIONS! YOU GOT the gastric balloon and have taken an important step towards losing weight!

The first few days can be a little rough. You may still feel some discomfort from getting the balloon system, and your body will still be getting used to the feeling of the balloon in your stomach. Plus, you'll be on a liquid diet, which is a challenge in itself.

Hang in there! These days will pass, and you will be on your way to losing weight and living healthy.

What to Expect

The procedure takes less than 30 minutes. After the doctor has filled the balloon system and checked to make sure it is not leaking, you will be released to go home. You will probably need to take it easy for about three days as you recover and adjust to the balloon being in your stomach.

You may feel some discomfort in the first few days or weeks after getting the balloon. Vomiting and nausea are especially common. Diarrhea, constipation, indigestion, and a feeling of fullness are also common. You can also get cramps or feel bloated. These are probably not medically serious, but you should always call your doctor if you are worried.

When to Contact Your Doctor

Most of the symptoms will go away within a few days or weeks, but some may be more serious. You should call your doctor if you think you may have more serious symptoms.

You should call your doctor immediately if you suspect a leak anytime the balloon system is in your stomach. You may have a leak if you suddenly feel that there is a loss of pressure or less of a feeling of fullness in your stomach. Some types of balloon systems contain a blue dye. If you see blue in your urine, you will know you have a leak.

What to Eat

This is the beginning of your time with the balloon. It is your chance to start fresh and establish good eating patterns that will help you through the next several months.

You're going to be pretty sore from getting the balloon system, so you will not be able to eat solid foods right away. Instead, you will start with liquids and then move to soft foods. This gives your throat and stomach a chance to heal after the procedure to insert the balloon.

Clear Liquid Diet

You might follow a clear liquid diet for the first day or two after getting the balloon. A clear liquid diet includes the following:

- Water

- Flavored water, such as Propel Fitness Water, Dasani Drops, and Crystal Light

- Diet sports drinks, such as G2 and Powerade Zero

- Decaffeinated coffee and tea

- Clear broth and bouillon

Avoid very hot and very cold drinks. Also, skip the carbonated beverages, including sparkling water and soft drinks.

Aim for 64 ounces (Eight 8-ounce cups) of liquid per day to prevent dehydration. Practice sipping slowly, and drink only about 1/3 to ½ cup of liquid at one time.

Full Liquid Diet

In a day or two, you can begin your full liquid diet. The full liquid diet helps you transition from clear liquids to solid foods. You can have all the liquids from the clear liquid diet, plus the following:

- Cream soups
- Watered down fruit juice
- Vegetable juice
- Pudding
- Low-sugar protein shakes

Be sure to ask your doctor about the exact foods you can have at this stage. You may be able to include yogurt, watery cream of wheat and strained oatmeal, and smooth mashed potatoes and sweet potatoes.

Keep drinking plenty of liquids to avoid dehydration and keep your energy levels up.

Liquids for Your Long-Term Success

Naturally, you think about fluids a lot during the first few days with the gastric balloon, since you're on a liquid diet. Once you are eating solid foods again, it's easy to let fluids fall to the wayside. After all, they're just...*there*...right?

Wrong!

Why Water? Weight Loss and More!

Food choices tend to get most of the attention when you're trying to lose weight, but what and how much you drink is just as important. Water can actually help you lose weight.

- It is like the miracle diet food of your dreams because it helps fill you up without giving you any calories.

- It prevents dehydration, which makes you feel tired. When you stay hydrated and energized, you can move around more and burn more calories throughout the day.

- It supports healthy metabolism.

But wait ... there's more! Water also helps your overall health. It prevents dehydration headaches, allows your skin and lips to appear healthy rather than dry, and helps your body with temperature regulation. Drinking plenty of water may even reduce risk of urinary tract infections and certain cancers.

You need about 8 to 12 8-ounce cups of water a day. That's about the amount in 4 to 6 standard water bottles. If you're having trouble remembering to drink your water, make an effort to have a full water bottle on hand throughout the day. Start the day with some water, and keep your bottle with you in the car, at work, and at the gym.

Introducing Water: Your New Weight-Loss Buddy

You do not need to depend on plain water to hit your fluid needs. If you don't like plain water, or you want to mix up your options a little, you can make your water a little more interesting and try other beverages. Just make sure they're calorie-free or very low in calories, with no more than 5 to 10 calories a serving.

If you don't like plain water, give ice water a try. You may be surprised by how much more drinkable it is. You can also try jazzing up your water with wedges of lemon or lime, a slice or two of strawberry or peach, or some fresh mint or basil leaves.

These are some alternatives to water that are also low-calorie:

- Water-flavoring powders, such as Crystal Light and G2 powder

- Water-flavoring drops, such as Mio Water Enhancement, Dasani Drops, and Powerade Zero Drops

- Sugar-free Kool-Aid

- Diet iced teas, such as Arizona, Snapple, or Lipton

- Flavored water, such as Propel Zero, Nestle PureLife Splash, and VitaminWater

- Diet soft drinks[10]

- Decaffeinated green or black tea

- Decaffeinated coffee

Liquids and Sugar – Watch Out!

A liquid diet may seem good for weight loss, but that actually depends on your choices. One of the biggest mistakes you can make on your liquid diet and beyond is to get too much sugar from liquids.

---

10   While diet soft drinks do not contain calories or sugar, they still may not be healthy choices. Some research suggests they may drive up insulin levels and leave you feeling hungrier than you were before. People who drink diet sodas do not seem to lose more weight than those who drink regular sodas, so your best bet may be to avoid all sodas.

Consider this: sweetened beverages are the greatest source of added sugars in the typical American's diet. Furthermore, the average adult gets more than one-fifth of their total daily calories from beverages. Some sugar-sweetened drinks can have 100 or more calories per 8-ounce cup, or several hundred calories in a large order.

Don't be a victim! Be careful during the liquid diet phases and beyond to make sure beverages don't sabotage your efforts. Take in just one or a few sugary drinks a day, and you could be at risk for stopping your weight loss.

Watch out for these beverages because of their calories:

- Flavored milk, such as chocolate or strawberry milk

- Regular sports drinks

- Sugar-sweetened iced tea, hot tea, or iced or hot coffee drinks

- Milk-based coffee drinks such as cappuccinos, mochas, and lattes

- Alcoholic beverages such as wine, beer, and mixed drinks

Some drinks have calories, but also some beneficial nutrients. They are okay choices sometimes, but be sure to count the calories. Examples include:

- Skim milk and unsweetened soy milk, which have protein, calcium, and other nutrients

- Unsweetened almond and cashew milk, which have calcium and other nutrients

- 100 percent fruit juice, which has antioxidants but a lot of sugar

Transitioning from Liquids to Solids

After a few weeks, you still may be feeling a little sore from getting the balloon, so it's not yet time to move to a full solid foods diet. Instead, spend a few days or even a couple weeks eating softer foods. Focus on soft, healthy choices, such as:

- Oatmeal

- Well-cooked vegetables, such as carrots, green beans

- Very soft fruit, such as ripe bananas and cantaloupe

- Canned tuna

- Eggs

- Non-fat cottage cheese and yogurt

- Mashed sweet potatoes

- Canned beans and fat-free refried beans

- Tofu

- All-natural deli meat

- Avocados

- Lean ground turkey

You may not yet be ready for fibrous, stringy, or crunchy foods, such as:

- Salad and other raw vegetables

- Cooked, very fibrous vegetables such as asparagus and broccoli stalks

- Skins, peels, and seeds, such as apple skin, zucchini peel, and seeds in peppers

- Oranges and grapefruit

- Nuts, peanuts, and seeds, either on their own or baked into breads

- Tough meat

Sugary and fatty foods can make you feel nauseous. At this time, you should also be avoiding unhealthy choices such as:

- Baked goods, such as cookies, pies, cakes, and muffins

- Refined grains such as white bread (including bagels), white rice, white pasta, and refined cereal

- Fatty processed meats, such as pepperoni, bacon, sausage, and salami

- Sugary drinks, including sodas, juice drinks, sweetened iced tea, and coffee drinks

- Fried foods, such as French fries, doughnuts, onion rings, and chicken

- Fast food, such as pizza, burgers, burritos, and fried rice

YOUR CHALLENGE

The first few days with the balloon can be uncomfortable, so you may not feel like doing much of anything. Still, there's one thing you can do to help yourself now and later: get enough fluids.

So, your challenge is to get at least 64 ounces of clear fluids every day while you are on the liquid diet (and hopefully beyond). Remember: 64 ounces is the same as eight 8-ounce cups, four 16-ounce water bottles (about half the standard size of a plastic bottle), or a half-gallon.

THE MEAL PLAN

Your goal now is to recover after getting the balloon. These meal plans can help. There is one you can follow at the beginning on the clear liquid diet, and another for when you progress to full liquids within few days.

Clear Liquid

Meal 1

Meal	Menu
Breakfast	1 cup apple juice 1 cup coffee with sugar or honey (optional)
Snack 1	1 ½ cup gelatin
Lunch	1 cup chicken broth 1 cup grape juice
Snack 2	1 frozen ice pop 1 bottle sports drink
Dinner	1 cup beef broth 1 cup apple juice ½ cup gelatin

Meal 2

Meal	Menu
Breakfast	1 cup cranberry juice 1 cup coffee (sweetened with sugar or honey, optional)
Snack	1 frozen ice pop 1 cup coffee
Lunch	1 cup vegetable broth ½ cup gelatin 1 cup pulp-free orange juice
Snack 2	2 ½ cup gelatin 1 cup iced tea (sweetened with sugar, optional)
Dinner	1 cup chicken broth 1 frozen ice pop 1 cup grape juice

Full Liquid

Meal 1

Meal	Menu
Breakfast	Pumpkin Shake: ✓ ½ cup pureed canned pumpkin ✓ ½ cup skim milk or soy milk ✓ ½ cup nonfat plain or no-sugar-added Greek yogurt ✓ 1 scoop of low-sugar vanilla or unflavored protein powder ✓ ½ teaspoon cinnamon ✓ ¼ teaspoon nutmeg ✓ Low-calorie sweetener to taste
Snack 1	½ cup unsweetened applesauce
Lunch	Pureed split pea soup: 1/4 of recipe: ✓ 1 quart low-sodium vegetable or chicken broth (optional: substitute some skim milk for broth) ✓ 1 tablespoon olive oil ✓ 1 cup split peas ✓ ½ cup barley ✓ 2 carrots, peeled and chopped ✓ 2 stalks celery, diced ✓ 1 onion, peeled and chopped ✓ Basil, thyme, salt, and black pepper to taste ✓ (optional) 1 cup tofu Cook ingredients for 2 hours; then puree
Snack 2	1 cup of pureed cooked carrots.
Dinner	1 cup low-fat cream of tomato soup 1 sugar-free or low-fat pudding cup 1 cup skim milk or soy milk

Meal 2

Meal	Menu
Breakfast	Peanut butter and banana smoothie: ✓ 1 banana ✓ 1 tablespoon peanut butter ✓ 1 cup almond milk ✓ ½ cup non-fat plain, or no-sugar-added vanilla Greek yogurt ✓ ½ teaspoon vanilla extract ✓ (optional) low-calorie sweetener to taste
Snack 1	1 cup pureed low-fat cream of mushroom soup.
Lunch	Tofu berry spinach smoothie: ✓ ½ cup soft tofu ✓ 2 cups fresh spinach leaves (can substitute kale) ✓ 1 cup fresh or frozen blueberries ✓ 1 cup fresh or frozen strawberries ✓ ¼ cup avocado ✓ (optional) low-calorie sweetener to taste
Snack 2	1 sugar free or low-fat pudding cup
Dinner	1 cup pureed lentil soup made with: ✓ ½ water and ½ yogurt ✓ 1 cup pureed, well-cooked vegetables such as carrots, green beans, or cauliflower ✓ 1 cup orange juice

Chapter 4

Food – What to Eat and How Much

WHEW! YOU MADE it through the toughest part – the first month. You should be starting to feel a lot more comfortable with the balloon in your stomach. If you stuck to the liquid diets and you're feeling good, you're ready to move on to real foods. You can also get back to work and regular activities, and maybe even add in some exercise.

But more about that later. For now, let's get a handle on the basics of a healthy diet. We've mentioned healthy eating already, and you know you need to eat healthy, but what is "healthy eating?" Which foods should you choose, and which are the trouble foods? And, what role do portion sizes play, and what size portions should you have?

And, since this is a time to establish new habits, maybe it's time to talk about new strategies to replace the eating you have done for reasons other than hunger. In this chapter, we'll discuss:

1. What you can eat

   A. Good foods

   B. Bad foods

   C. Beverages

2. Challenge: Implement alternative strategies to avoid emotional eating, or boredom eating. We'll show you how to write down when they happen, what you would normally do (eat) and what you chose to do instead.

"What" to Eat: Good Foods and Bad Foods

What are good foods and bad foods? Which foods should you aim to have with your balloon and beyond, and which should you avoid? Why does it matter?

"Good" foods are "good" for a number of reasons.

- They're not just good for your overall health. They're also good for long-term weight loss and maintenance.

- They tend to be more filling with fewer calories compared to junk food.

- They stop your blood sugar from spiking and dropping, so you don't crave sugar or get super hungry.

- They hold your energy levels stable so you feel better and can be more active and burn more calories. You can feel better and lose more weight long term when you focus on "good" foods.

The Good Foods: Stock Your Kitchen

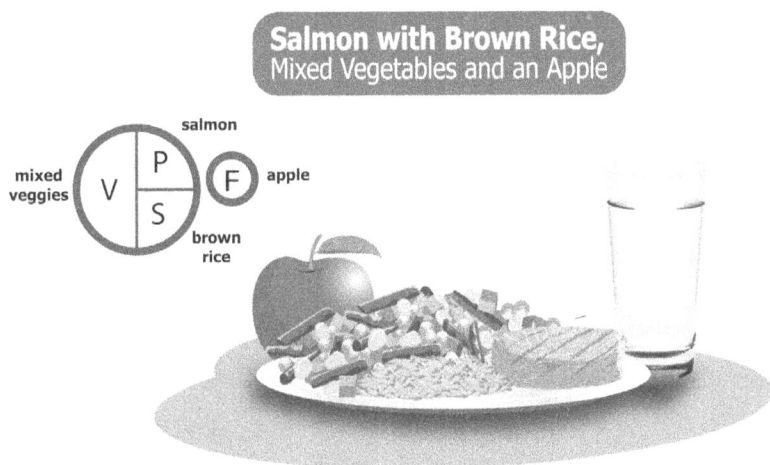

Salmon with Brown Rice, Mixed Vegetables and an Apple

The "good" foods tend to be less processed and more nutritious. They're better for weight loss because they're more satisfying, and they're less likely to trigger cravings for sugary, fatty foods. So what are these "good" foods? They're the ones we discussed in Chapter 2 under protein, carbs, and fats.

Here are the basics.

- **Non-starchy vegetables.** These are the foundation of your diet.

- **Lean proteins,** such as fish, beans, eggs, reduced-fat dairy products, soy products and tofu, chicken, nuts and turkey. A serving should be in most meals and snacks.

- **Legumes, or beans, peas, and lentils.** They're a superstar cross of lean protein and high-fiber starch.

- **Whole grains and starchy vegetables.** They're high-fiber, high-nutrient, and energy-providing.

- **Fruit.** Choose it instead of sugary treats, and you're doing well!

- **Healthy fats**. Keep portions small, but keep them in your diet.

You can see food lists in Appendix A.

Bad Foods: Okay as a Treat

You do not need to avoid all "bad" foods all the time. The healthiest way to approach them is to have them occasionally. It is okay if there is a certain food you cannot live without, such as brownies or pizza.

Just plan for it as an occasional treat. You can still lose weight if you have a piece of cake for your birthday and exercise afterward. You'll have a much tougher time losing weight if you have half a pizza for dinner and a large slice of cake with ice cream for dessert every day.

You can also keep some of those favorite foods in your diet by planning for them. If you know ahead of time you will want to indulge, you can work your treat into your meal plans. It could be a few drinks with friends, dinner at a restaurant, or your favorite dessert, for example. Estimate the calories, and plan for them by lowering your calories for the rest of the day.

You might even consider getting in a workout before or after the treat. Along with burning a few extra calories, it'll keep you focused on your weight-loss goal. It can help you feel good about your treat and ready to move on, rather than out of control about "caving in."

Day-to-day, you can work in your treats by making them smaller or substituting similar foods. These are some examples.

- Go for pureed cauliflower instead of buttery mashed potatoes (save 200 calories).

- Make homemade pizza on portabella mushroom instead of ordering in and having a few slices (save 500 calories).

- Have a ½ cup of frozen yogurt and fill your bowl with berries instead having a large bowl of regular ice cream (save 300 calories).

- Satisfy chocolate cravings with a fudge pop, or sugar-free hot chocolate made with unsweetened almond milk, instead of a brownie or chocolate cake (save 300 calories).

- Get your crunch on with veggies and fat-free spinach artichoke dip made with non-fat cream cheese instead of downing chips and full-fat dip.

You can often fit treats regularly into your diet by watching the portion sizes and eating them as part of a lower-calorie meal or snack. These are some examples.

- You can start your day off okay if you stick to a half-piece of coffee cake from a bakery for 200 calories, and add ½ cup of cottage cheese plus a serving of fruit.

- A slice of pizza for 200 calories plus a side salad makes for a reasonable lunch.

- You can come in under 500 calories for dinner if you have some chicken or fish, a vegetable, and a small iced brownie for 300 calories.

- Sneak in an ounce of tortilla chips and some salsa for a 200-calorie snack.

These are not the healthiest of choices, but they can satisfy cravings so you can go back to your healthy eating patterns without seeing a blip on the scale.

Why Does the "What" Matter?

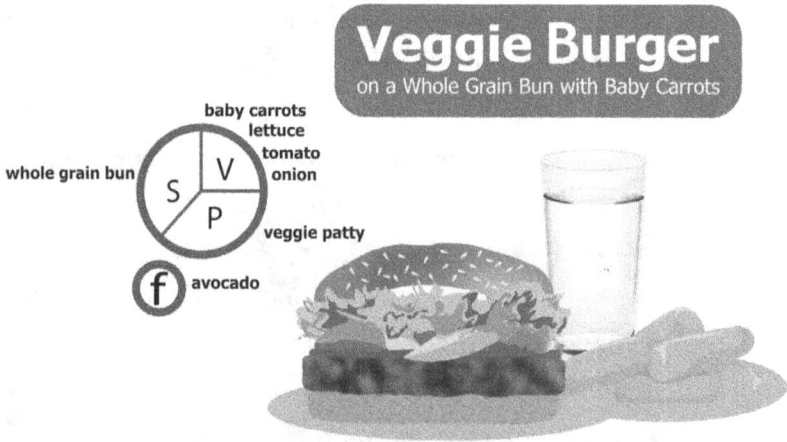

Veggie Burger
on a Whole Grain Bun with Baby Carrots

whole grain bun — baby carrots / lettuce / tomato / onion — veggie patty — avocado

It's true you can lose weight eating pretty much anything. Every so often, you might run across a story in the news about someone who lost weight eating only at McDonald's or loading up on Twinkies.

If calories in versus calories out determines weight loss, why does "what" you eat matter? A couple of the major reasons are sustainability and health.

You can lose weight by eating a doughnut (300 calories) for breakfast, a small hamburger and fries (500 calories) for lunch, and a slice of pepperoni pizza with a cookie (500 calories) for dinner. That menu adds up to a total of 1,300 calories.

But this meal plan probably isn't sustainable. It's likely to leave you hungry day after day because of the sugar from the doughnut and cookie, refined carbs from the doughnut, burger bun, fries, and pizza, and saturated fat from the doughnut, burger patty, and pizza. Sugar, refined carbs, and saturated fat drive up blood sugar. When blood sugar later plummets, you can feel starving even though you just ate an hour or so ago.

Pretty soon, you'll probably get sick of feeling hungry nearly all the time, and go off your "diet." In this case, you're most likely to add in extra food to satisfy hunger, and you'll bump up your calories. That's one reason why this unhealthy diet isn't sustainable.

Another reason is that sugars, refined carbs, and fatty, salty foods can all be addictive. The more pizza, doughnuts, and fries you eat, the more you want. Your brain will be asking for more of these unhealthy foods, and you're likely to cave in eventually.

Beyond weight loss, these foods are also bad for general health. Too much of them can increase risk for heart disease, diabetes, and even Alzheimer's disease. They can increase cancer risk. When you choose them instead of healthy foods, you can get vitamin and mineral deficiencies even if you are eating a lot of calories.

On the other hand, when your meal plan depends mostly on healthy foods, you have fewer cravings, less hunger, and lower risk for serious medical conditions in the long term.

The "How Much" Matters, Too: Portion Control and the Balloon

It's not just "what" you eat that matters. "How much" you eat affects weight loss just as much. The balloon is designed to help you control your portions. It helps you feel full sooner, so you eat less. Not as much food fits in your stomach.

These are some proper serving sizes to think about when you serve yourself.

Food and Serving Size	Looks Like...
3 ounces cooked chicken, ground turkey, fish, and lean meat	✓ Deck of cards ✓ A checkbook
½ cup cooked beans, rice, or oatmeal ½ cup cooked vegetables ½ cup cottage cheese	½ a baseball or tennis ball
1 cup cooked pasta or breakfast cereal 1 cup of cut fruit or raw vegetables A medium apple or orange	A tennis ball or baseball
1 ounce of cheese	Four stacked dice
1 tablespoon of peanut butter or oil	The upper portion of your thumb
1 small bagel or English muffin or a slice of bread	A hockey puck
1 teaspoon of margarine	Your thumbnail
2 tablespoons of salad dressing	A ping-pong ball

Portions Are Out of Control!

If some of the serving sizes you just read seem small, it may be because we are living in a world of oversized portions! Many foods and beverages often come in double, triple, or even bigger sizes compared against what you *should* be having. These are just a few examples of such oversized portions.

- Large fries: 6 servings.
- Muffin or bagel from a coffee shop or bakery: 5 servings.
- Plate of pasta from a restaurant: 5 servings.
- Jumbo soft pretzel: 4 servings.
- Large sub sandwich: 4 servings.
- Large baked potato: 3 servings.
- Bottle of soda or juice: 2.5 servings.
- Double hamburger: 2 servings.

You can protect yourself by being aware of what you *need* versus what you are *served.* You never need to eat the entire plate. You can put away the extras before you start eating and save them for later, or throw away the leftovers when you are full. It is better to waste food by throwing it away than to waste it by eating it and letting it sit in your body as fat.

Measuring cups and spoons can help you get exact portion sizes. A digital or analog food scale is another useful tool. Even if you're pretty sure about your estimates, it's a good idea to measure your foods exactly, especially at the beginning. You may be surprised that your estimates weren't perfect!

You can find healthy food lists in Appendix A.

Learning to Recognize Fullness with the Balloon

The big benefit of the balloon is that it helps you feel full sooner by slowing digestion and taking up space in your stomach. While the balloon is in your stomach, take the opportunity to learn how to recognize fullness. Notice how hungry you are when you start to eat, and stop eating when you first begin to get full. You should stop eating when you are just barely full, and not when you are stuffed or even satisfied.

Your brain takes a while to recognize when you are no longer hungry. It takes about 20 minutes or more for your stomach to send signals to your brain that you are full. So, you should make sure to take at least 20 minutes to eat each meal before you even think about going for seconds.

To slow down your eating, you can:

- Chew your food at least 30 times, or until it is completely mushy in your mouth.

- Put down your fork between bites.

- Think about tasting each bite and noticing the flavors, textures, and smells.

- Talk a lot if you are eating with other people.

- Serve yourself on smaller dishes so you take less.

- Do not allow yourself to serve yourself seconds until at least 20 minutes pass.

- Use smaller forks and spoons.

- Try using chopsticks or eating with your left hand.

Mindful Eating

Mindful eating is good habit that can help you eat more slowly and eat less overall. Research suggests that people who practice mindful eating may be able to lose more weight. Mindful eating simply means paying attention to what you eat instead of eating without thinking about it.

Practice asking yourself a few questions every time you eat.

- *Am I hungry?* You may be eating a surprisingly high amount of food when you are not even hungry. What a waste of calories when you are trying to lose weight!

- *What is triggering me to want to eat now?* Hunger is a great reason to eat. Habit is not. Neither are convenience, stress, or boredom.

- *What do I feel like eating?* You may just be reaching for whatever is there or whatever you are used to without consciously choosing it. That is unfortunate if you're used to grabbing cookies or chips, when your body is really asking for some sweet grapes or crunchy carrots!

- *Am I enjoying this food's taste, texture, and smell?* Notice your food and appreciate it so you can get the full satisfaction you deserve.

- *Why did I just eat that?* You may forget to be mindful while you are eating, but you can always learn from your mistakes. Instead of getting mad at yourself for overeating, try to figure out why it happened so it does not need to happen again.

In most cases, there is an underlying reason that is causing poor food decisions and overeating. Figure out what the underlying reason is and address that reason. That will be far more effective in the long term than just looking at the overeating – or end result of that underlying reason. At the same time, you can work on finding alternatives to overeating when you do get stressed, bored, or in another trigger situation.

Emotional or Stress Eating: If you're an emotional eater, you use food to comfort you or make you feel better. Binges can be triggered by stressful events, frustration, good news, bad news, and loneliness. It takes work, but it is possible to conquer emotional eating.

- Learn to recognize when you are eating for emotional comfort versus for hunger.

- Try to reduce stress. Healthy strategies involve regularly exercising, taking time to relax or meditate, getting enough sleep, and talking over your anxieties with a friend or family member.

- Keep "binge" foods out of the house, or at least hard to access. For example, don't keep ice cream in the freezer if that's your typical go-to. And if mashed potatoes are one of your triggers, don't keep leftovers on hand. You're far less likely to eat your trigger foods if they're not staring you in the face.

Learn to recognize, accept, and embrace your emotions. Emotional eaters often use food as a way to escape feelings. Guess what: if you actually learn to feel your feelings, you may find they're not as bad as you feared. Start to appreciate being able to feel positive and negative emotions. They can tell you a lot, and you can be proud of yourself when you address the causes of those feelings rather than running away.

Boredom Eating

You take a handful of nuts when you walk through the kitchen, you munch on a bowl of popcorn while you're watching TV, you always have a protein bar stashed in the car, you taste whatever you're cooking for dinner while you're still in the kitchen, and you snack on cheese and apples when you're doing the chores.

In short, you're snacking throughout the day.

This boredom eating, mindless munching, or grazing can leave you with too many calories, but it's a hard habit to give up. Focus on distracting yourself. Get engaged in the moment so you don't feel the need for food to fill a void. Focus more on other people and on the task at hand.

Also, boredom eaters, possibly even more than other people, can benefit from food logging. When you actually log each bite, you may be shocked that your little "tastes" add up to hundreds of calories a day. You may realize it's just not worth it!

Logging can also help you visualize the damage you're doing when you sneak a bite here and there. It can motivate you to not take that extra bite or handful or serving. When you visualize adding the calories to your food log, logging can also motivate you to choose the lower-calorie options. You might skip a few hundred calories of, say, dried fruit in favor of a stack of cucumber slices for 20 calories.

Finally, tune in to your hunger cues to break the habit of eating for entertainment. Learn to stop yourself from grabbing food when you're not really hungry. Ask, "Am I hungry or am I bored?" You can get in the habit of not taking the food when the answer is, "I'm bored."

Depression Eating

Depression can also lead to poor eating habits. It can feel embarrassing, but there's no shame in getting help for depression. Together with a mental health professional and the support of your trusted friends or family members, you can work to deal with depression. It may involve medications, behavior change such as more exercise, coping strategies, or some combination of those options.

Getting a handle on depression will leave you with more energy and better able to make healthy eating choices.

Food Tracking: A Powerful Tool

Research overwhelmingly shows the power of logging the food you eat. Logging:

- Helps keep you accountable so you do not lie to yourself.

- Helps you make healthier decisions because you're more likely to choose the "right" foods and portions if you know you're going to be recording them later.

- Helps you figure out what you can improve on by showing you surprisingly high values for calories or certain nutrients.

There are so many tools available for logging. Experiment a little, and choose the one that works best for you. The best tool:

- Is easy and quick, so you feel like doing it.

- Tells you the values you need, such as calories, protein, or fiber.

- Lets you record any other information you want, such as weight or activity.

You can log your food the old-fashioned way with a pen and paper journal, or go a little higher tech with a web-based site or mobile app. Electronic food journals usually have a large database of foods, and let you enter your own foods and recipes. You can usually add extra information like activity, weight, and body measurements.

Another nice feature of electronic journals is their memory. You can check what you ate last week and last month, and usually you can see graphs and charts showing your trends over time, whether you're interested in calories, protein, fiber, or even certain vitamins and minerals.

Download a mobile app, and you can get all the great features you're looking for on the go. Log your meals as soon as you eat them wherever you are. Check calorie counts of certain foods, including restaurant foods, before you make your final decision. It takes only seconds, and that convenience may be what keeps you faithful to your food logging intentions and your diet.

You can also go social with your food logging. Join a group and open your food diary to friends, and you can motivate each other, trade recipes, and talk about strategies, challenges, and successes.

Start with the Basics

Get too ambitious at the beginning, and you might get overwhelmed or frustrated or give up on food logging before it becomes a habit. Before you worry about too many details, just focus on getting the basics down.

Log each food and the amount you eat. Since calories are the most important part of your weight-loss plan, check your daily calories to make sure they're within your goal range.

Once you're comfortable with logging foods and checking calories, you can think about moving on to tracking more nutrients, but only if you want to. You can look at your protein, carbs, fat, and fiber. You can check servings of vegetables, fruits, and protein. You can compare calories consumed with calories burned. You can look at your ratios of saturated to unsaturated fats. You can get as detailed as you like ... but don't feel pressure to track everything.

Beyond the Balloon

You'll be working to keep portion sizes down the whole time you have the balloon and beyond. Food choices and portion sizes are your keys to losing weight and keeping it off for the long haul. You have a while until you need to think about eating without the balloon, but you can be confident that the skills you're working on now will help you be successful in the long run, including after you get the balloon system deflated and taken out.

YOUR CHALLENGE

Your challenge is to practice two behaviors that can kick weight loss up a notch. So, there are two challenges for you this month!

The first is to measure your food. See if you can measure every bite of food at least 5 days out of the week. Measuring so consistently can help you make it a habit. It can also help you get used to the proper-sized portions so you can get the right amount of food even when you're somewhere where you can't measure, such as at a restaurant.

Your second challenge is to stop eating just before you're full. This is a tough one, but it is worth practicing. You may have trouble figuring out the sweet spot at first, but keep trying. When you stop eating just before you're full, you learn to leave the table before you're overstuffed. The payoff? Big weight loss! See if you can stop eating before you're full at least 10 times in the next week.

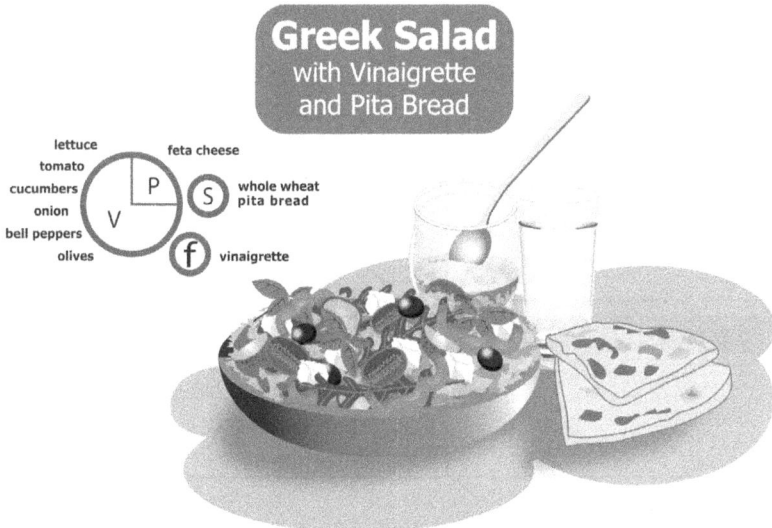

Greek Salad
with Vinaigrette
and Pita Bread

lettuce
tomato
cucumbers
onion
bell peppers
olives

feta cheese

P

S

V

f

whole wheat
pita bread

vinaigrette

THE MEAL PLAN

Each meal plan includes foods that you can have on a soft diet, and each day has about 1,200 calories.

Remember, you can switch around the foods on the plan to allow for extra snacks;for example, if you wanted, you could have the cantaloupe listed below for a morning snack instead of having it with dinner.

Meal 1

Meal	Menu
Breakfast	Cheesy scrambled eggs made with: ✓ 2 eggs ✓ 1 ounce low-fat cheese, such as mozzarella or cheddar ✓ 2 tablespoons milk or almond milk ✓ Oatmeal made with ½ cup oats and 1 cup almond milk
Lunch	Couscous salad with veggies: ✓ 1/3 cup dry whole wheat couscous, prepared using water or low-sodium chicken or vegetable broth ✓ 1 cup cooked diced vegetables, such as zucchini, bell peppers, onions, carrots, or green beans ✓ 2 teaspoons olive oil ✓ Black pepper, fresh basil leaves, and lemon juice to taste ✓ 1 cup ripe cantaloupe in cubes
Dinner	4 ounces baked halibut with 1 teaspoon olive oil, lemon juice, and salt and pepper to taste. 1 medium sweet potato, baked 1 cup cooked cauliflower ½ cup fat-free frozen yogurt

Meal 2

Meal	Menu
Breakfast	Overnight pumpkin oatmeal – stir together the night before: ✓ ½ cup oats ✓ ¼ cup fat-free milk or unsweetened almond milk ✓ ¼ cup canned pumpkin puree ✓ ½ teaspoon cinnamon ✓ 1-2 packets low-calorie sweetener 1 cup of fruit salad with cut fruit or berries, such as cut melon, apples, or pears, or grapes, blueberries, strawberries, or blackberries.
Lunch	¼ recipe minestrone stew made with: ✓ 1 cup low-sodium beef or vegetable broth ✓ 1 diced carrot ✓ 2 stalks diced celery ✓ ½ diced onion ✓ 2 cloves garlic ✓ One 8-ounce can tomato sauce ✓ 1 large diced tomato ✓ 1 can kidney beans ✓ 1 can garbanzo beans ✓ ½ cup cooked barley ✓ 1 cup cooked green beans ✓ Basil, oregano, and pepper Serve with your choice of 1-ounce crumbled blue cheese (or another kind of cheese), or 3 ounces cooked diced chicken breast. 1 medium apple 1 tablespoon peanut butter

Meal	Menu
Dinner	¼ recipe turkey meatloaf: ✓ 1 pound (16 ounces) lean ground turkey ✓ ½ cup each of grated onion, grated zucchini, and grated carrots ✓ ½ cup Italian seasoned canned tomatoes ✓ 1 egg ✓ ½ cup oats ✓ 1 packet spaghetti sauce seasoning mix or onion soup mix ½ cup mashed potatoes made with milk, nutmeg, and 1 tablespoon parmesan cheese ¼ recipe watermelon corn salsa: ✓ 1 cup corn ✓ 1 cup watermelon ✓ 1 cup diced tomatoes ✓ 1 cup chopped cucumber ✓ ¼ onion, chopped and marinated in lime juice ✓ Fresh cilantro leaves ✓ Garlic powder, red pepper flakes, and black pepper to taste ✓ (optional) 1 packet of low-calorie sweetener

Chapter 5

Meal Planning and Exercise: Critical for Success

AS YOU ENTER the second month, you should be getting a little more comfortable with the feeling of the balloon in your stomach. You're eating healthy, watching your portions, and losing a bit of weight. Life's good!

Now that you're getting used to choosing healthy foods and eating the right amount, you can get a little deeper into the process. It's time to take what you know already, and apply it to meal planning. We'll go over how to make healthy meals and menus that fit your calorie and nutrient goals and keep you on track for satisfying weight loss.

It's also a good time now to think about exercise. Getting active can help you lose weight, feel energized, and stay motivated to eat well. People who successfully maintain their weight loss over the long term are often the same people who make exercise a regular part of their day.

From Foods to Meals and Menus

You can already recognize the list of healthy foods you should be choosing. Can you also put those foods together and create healthy meals and daily menus? Here's your chance to learn!

From Foods to Meals

Your meals and snacks may be smaller with the balloon than they used to be. A meal may consist of something like one or two servings of vegetables or fruit, *plus* a serving of protein, *plus* one or two servings of healthy starch or fat. For example:

- Vegetable plus protein and starch: Broiled salmon plus roasted asparagus and sweet potato.

- Fruit plus protein and starch: Berries plus oatmeal made with skim milk.

- Vegetable plus protein and healthy fat: mixed green salad with sliced hard-boiled eggs and olive oil vinaigrette.

A snack may include a protein *plus* a vegetable, fruit, healthy fat, or starch. For example:

- A protein plus a vegetable: non-fat cream cheese plus celery.

- A protein plus fruit: non-fat cottage cheese plus apple slices.

- A protein plus healthy fat: mixed nuts.

- A protein plus a starch: half a whole-grain English muffin plus all-natural low-sodium turkey.

Appendix A shows which foods belong to which food group. You can check what counts as a protein, vegetable, fruit, starch, and fat.

From Meals to Menus

You can put a few meals and snacks together to build your daily meal plan or menu. While you're working with your doctor and nutritionist, they may give you the goal to get 1,000 to 1,200 calories each day. You can do this by eating three meals, or by breaking it up into three small meals plus two snacks.

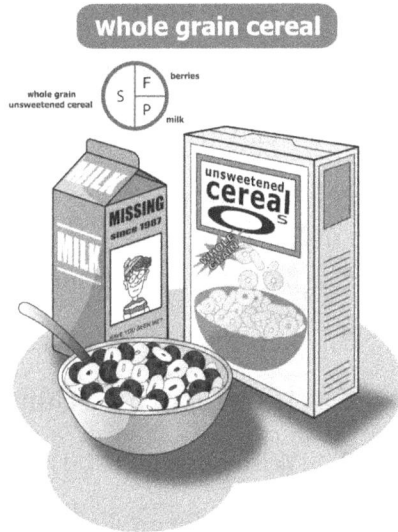

whole grain cereal

You can build your menus by putting together some meals and, if you want, one or two snacks. If you're aiming for three meals per day without snacks, each meal should have 300 to 400 calories.

Here's a sample day:

Breakfast (300 calories):

- 2 small whole-grain pancakes (2 starches)
- 1 scrambled egg (1 protein)
- 1 cup blueberries (1 fruit)

Lunch (500 calories):

- 1 small whole-grain tortilla or wrap (1 starch)
- ½ cup fat-free refried beans (1 protein)
- 1 ounce low-fat shredded cheese (1 protein)
- 1 ounce avocado (1 fat)
- 1 cup grilled vegetables (2 vegetables)

Dinner (400 calories)

- 3 ounces lean ground turkey (1 protein)
- Lettuce leaves as a wrap, plus tomatoes (1 vegetable)
- 1 cup roasted zucchini sticks (1 vegetable)
- With olive oil (1 fat)
- 1 medium apple (1 fruit)

Total: 1,200 calories

If you're going for three meals and two snacks a day, aim for 250 to 300 calories at mealtimes, plus 100 to 200 calories per snack. Your day could look like this.

Breakfast (250 calories):

- Scrambled eggs made with 1 egg, 2 egg whites, and 1 cup of chopped broccoli (2 protein plus 1 vegetable)
- ½ whole-grain English muffin (1 starch)

Snack 1 (150 calories):

- 1 cup plain non-fat yogurt (1 protein)
- 1 cup strawberries (1 fruit)

Lunch (300 calories):

- 2 cups romaine lettuce (1 vegetable)
- 1 cup raw vegetables such as mushrooms, tomatoes, cucumbers, and bell peppers (1 vegetable)
- 3 ounces grilled skinless chicken breast (1 protein)
- 2 tablespoons olive oil and herb vinaigrette (1 fat)

Snack 2 (200 calories):

- 1 ounce almonds (1 protein/fat)
- 1 cup cherry tomatoes

Dinner (300 calories)

- 3 ounces broiled halibut (1 protein)
- 1 medium sweet potato (1 starch)
- 1 ounce sliced avocado (1 fat)

Total: 1200 calories

Remember, start with healthy foods and a balanced variety, and your daily menus will turn out healthy and balanced.

Striving for the Perfect Balance: How to Adjust to Hit Your Calorie Goals

If you find you need more or fewer calories than the amount in the meal plans or daily food group patterns, just tweak them to meet your needs.

Even if you need to add calories to hit your goals, you do not want to add empty calories from junk food. Adding sugary foods or a soda, cooking eggs or smothering your bread with butter, and downing a bag of potato chips will get you calories, but it's not a healthy way to go. Instead, think about adding nutrient-dense foods. Often, healthy fats such as nuts are good choices.

You can always add calories by increasing the portion size of one or more foods. You could also add an extra food or another serving of a food that you're already having to a meal or snack. You can even add in an extra snack to hit your goals.

These are some easy examples of how you can add some nutritious calories:

- Add avocado to a salad or soup
- Spread hummus on your bread or wrap
- Snack on nuts or edamame
- Add barley, split peas, lentils, or beans to soup

Other times, you may need to cut out calories from a meal. You shouldn't need to do it much when following the plans in this book, because they are designed for balloon patients. Still, there will be other times when you'll want to cut a few calories.

This is harder than adding calories, but you can do it! You can take smaller portions, eat only certain parts of the meal, and choose lower-calorie swaps for higher-calorie foods. These are some examples:

- Pack up half your restaurant meal before starting to eat.
- Order your toppings as a salad on a bed of lettuce, rather than a sandwich or wrap on bread or a tortilla.
- Skip the butter and mayo.
- Get light instead of regular dressing.
- Eat only the burger patty or grilled chicken breast, and not the bun.
- Serve yourself an extra helping of vegetables, and skip the starchy potatoes, pasta, or rice.
- Serve yourself less cereal and more fruit.

Here's another guide to help you plan meals. Every day on a 1,000 to 1,200-calorie diet, you should aim to get in the following:

- 3-5 servings of vegetables

- 2-3 servings of fruit

- 3-4 servings of protein

- 2-4 servings of healthy grains or starches

- 2 servings of healthy fats

Eat Your Veggies – No Problem!

Vegetables are the foundation of your gastric balloon weight-loss diet. They take up space and fill you up without adding many calories. They're high in fiber to keep you full for longer, and they have all kinds of powerful nutrients.

You're in luck if you already know how to pack in the vegetables, but even if you don't, there's no need to despair! It's easy to get the three, five, or even more servings of veggies you need every day.

Snack Veggies

Need a quick snack? Reach for fresh vegetables. Some veggies are great on their own, and some are perfect for dipping. You can even use veggies to make your dip! All of these are good snack options.

- Grape tomatoes, baby carrots, and sugar snap peas

- Celery with non-fat cream cheese

- Cucumber with Greek yogurt and dill

- Carrot sticks with ranch dip made with Greek yogurt and a dry ranch flavoring packet

- Baked kale chips with olive oil and salt and pepper or parmesan cheese

- Whole-wheat crackers or bell pepper strips with dip made with pureed eggplant dip with cooked eggplant, garlic, lemon, tahini, and salt

- Raw cauliflower florets dipped into pureed pea dip with curry seasoning

Side and Center Veggies

Make your meal bigger and more filling by adding vegetables. They go with almost everything! Have them on the side, or cook them right into the main dish.

- Scrambled eggs and omelets with spinach and mushrooms, tomatoes and onions, peppers and corn, or zucchini.

- Add a side of steamed vegetables such as broccoli, cauliflower, zucchini, or Brussels sprouts, or roasted veggies such as carrots, turnips, onions, or cabbage.

- Have a side salad or main course salad with lettuce, raw veggies, and your choice of protein.

- Add lettuce, sprouts, tomatoes, and onions to sandwiches, or go a little fancier and add grilled or roasted vegetables such as bell pepper and eggplant.

- Add your favorites to soup, stew, and spaghetti sauce.

- Think of stir fry as a veggie dish with a ton of veggies and a little protein.

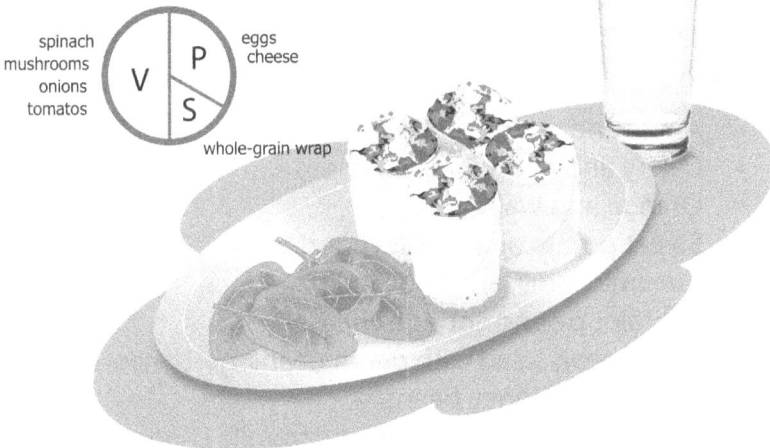

Veggie Egg Wraps
with Spinach Leaves

spinach
mushrooms
onions
tomatos

V
P
S

eggs
cheese

whole-grain wrap

Sneaky Veggies

If you're still not a fan of veggies, you can get them in sneakier ways. You can get your filling fiber without even realizing it!

- Fruit and yogurt smoothies with kale, spinach, canned pumpkin, and cucumber.

- Add extra spaghetti sauce to pizza and pasta.

- Add pureed cooked cauliflower and winter squash to tomato sauce.

- Grated zucchini, carrots, and eggplant in meatloaf.

Snack Time!

Snacks can reduce hunger so you're not starving by your next meal. When you keep hunger in check, you're less likely to dive for sugary, fatty foods or to eat way too fast or too much.

A snack should give you lasting energy, but some kinds of snacks do exactly the opposite. Get too much sugar, refined starch, or saturated fat, and you may be heading for a blood sugar spike and an energy crash in an hour. Healthy snacks boost your energy and stabilize blood sugar levels rather than spike them. You can put together healthy snacks by choosing a vegetable or a fruit and adding some protein. They can be pretty simple:

- Apple and peanut butter
- Celery and non-fat cream cheese
- Orange and walnuts
- Sweet potato and Greek yogurt
- Cucumber, dill, and yogurt dip
- Cantaloupe and cottage cheese
- Three-bean salad with green beans, garbanzo beans, and kidney beans
- Kebabs with chicken, tofu, mozzarella cheese, or shrimp, and vegetables or fruit

You can find all kinds of healthy snack ideas ranging from under 100 calories to over 200 calories in Appendix C.

Another Tool: The Nutrition Label

The nutrition label can be one of your biggest allies in the battle of the bulge. It can help you select foods at the grocery store and when cooking at home. The nutrition label tells you most of what you need to know. It has calories, and lists the protein, carbohydrate, and fat contents. It tells you the amount of saturated and trans fat, sodium, cholesterol, and fiber. The label may also show vitamin A, vitamin C, iron, and calcium.

This is a standard nutrition label for a hypothetical food: frozen bean and cheese enchiladas.

Nutrition Facts

Serving Size 1 Enchilada (140g)
Servings Per Container 2

Amount Per Serving

Calories 190   Calories from Fat 50

	% Daily Values*
Total Fat 7g	**11%**
Saturated Fat 2g	**10%**
Trans Fat 0g	
Cholesterol 120mg	**40%**
Sodium 400mg	**17%**
Total Carbohydrate 22g	**7%**
Dietary Fiber 5g	**20%**
Sugars 3g	
Protein 8g	**16%**

Vitamin A 10%	•		Vitamin C 6%
Calcium 15%	•		Iron 20%

*Percent Daily Values are based on a 2,000 calorie diet. Your Daily Values may be higher or lower depending on your calorie needs.

	Calories	2,000	2,500
Total Fat	Less than	65g	80g
Sat Fat	Less than	20g	25g
Cholesterol	Less than	300mg	300mg
Sodium	Less than	2400mg	2400mg
Total Carbohydrate		300g	375g
Dietary Fiber		25g	30g

When you look at this label, you can see a lot of information to help you decide whether this is a good lunch for you.

- It has a reasonable number of calories – 190 – per serving. That can fit into your diet.

- It has a good amount of fat, with 50 calories from fat. That's 28 percent of the total calories, which fits in your meal plan.

- It has some protein and carbohydrates to balance out the fat.

- It is high in fiber.

- It's a good source of vitamin A, iron, and calcium.

- It has two servings per package – so watch out!

- It's high in sodium.

On the whole, this enchilada could be a good basis for a lunch or dinner, possibly with the addition of some veggies or a piece of fruit. It is calorie-controlled and balanced. Since it's so high in sodium, you might want to eat less salty, less processed foods the rest of the day.

Serving Size Matters!

Be sure to check the serving size. It may be smaller than you think. Often, you may expect the serving to be an entire package, but the nutrition label is for half or a third of the package. If you eat the whole package, you need to multiply by two or three. For example, if the serving size is half a burrito and each serving has 300 calories, you'll be getting 600 calories if you eat the whole burrito.

Here are some common foods that have tricky serving sizes:

- **Snack foods:** You may be tempted to eat the whole bag, but a bag can have multiple servings.

- **Cereal:** A serving may be as small as 1/3 of a cup if it's a dense cereal like granola.

- **Meats and poultry:** A "piece" of meat can be enough for several people, even if you intended to make it as a single dinner for you and your family.

- **Beverages:** A 20-ounce bottle of soda or sports drinks, and orders of coffee drinks and smoothies can have multiple servings according to the nutrition label, even though you're clearly intending to drink the entire thing at once.

- **Frozen meals:** You may assume they're "single-serving" meals, but they are often meant for two people.

Check the Ingredients

The label also has a list of ingredients in the food. The list of ingredients gives you a lot of good information. Know that the ingredients are listed in order of weight. The first ingredient is the ingredient with the biggest amount, followed by the second ingredient, and so forth. So, if you see a list that has, "flour, tomatoes, beef, and salt," you know there is more flour than anything else, and more tomatoes than beef and salt.

Here are some other things to look at when checking the ingredients:

- If you're choosing a grain, see if the main ingredients are whole grains, such as "whole wheat flour." If you simply see "wheat flour" without the word "whole," you know the product is not whole grain.

- Check for various kinds of sugars, such as sugar, white sugar, brown sugar, molasses, honey, corn syrup, high fructose corn syrup, cane juice, dextrose, and turbinado sugar. They all drive up your blood sugar and have calories.

- Avoid products with partially hydrogenated or fully hydrogenated oils. They have saturated or trans fats.

Choosing Between Products

The nutrition label can help you decide which product, food, or dish to choose. Let's say you're looking for a healthy, filling canned soup for lunch. You're deciding between two brands of split pea soup and want to know which is healthier.

Here are their labels.

Brand 1:

Nutrition Facts

Serving Size 1 Cup (256g)
Servings Per Container 2

Amount Per Serving

Calories 180   Calories from Fat 60

	% Daily Values*
Total Fat 7g	**11%**
Saturated Fat 4g	**20%**
Trans Fat 0g	
Cholesterol 30mg	**10%**
Sodium 670mg	**28%**
Total Carbohydrate 23g	**8%**
Dietary Fiber 4g	**16%**
Sugars 7g	
Protein 8g	**16%**

Vitamin A 4%   •   Vitamin C 2%

Iron 10%

*Percent Daily Values are based on a 2,000 calorie diet. Your Daily Values may be higher or lower depending on your calorie needs.

	Calories	2,000	2,500
Total Fat	Less than	65g	80g
Sat Fat	Less than	20g	25g
Cholesterol	Less than	300mg	300mg
Sodium	Less than	2400mg	2400mg
Total Carbohydrate		300g	375g
Dietary Fiber		25g	30g

Brand 2:

Nutrition Facts

Serving Size 1 Cup (258g)
Servings Per Container 2

Amount Per Serving

Calories 150   Calories from Fat 35

% Daily Values*

Total Fat 4g	**6%**
Saturated Fat 1g	**5%**
Trans Fat 0g	
Cholesterol 30mg	**10%**
Sodium 320mg	**13%**
Total Carbohydrate 20g	**7%**
Dietary Fiber 7g	**28%**
Sugars 3g	
Protein 12g	**24%**

Vitamin A 2%	•	Vitamin C 4%
Calcium 4%	•	Iron 15%

*Percent Daily Values are based on a 2,000 calorie diet. Your Daily Values may be higher or lower depending on your calorie needs.

	Calories	2,000	2,500
Total Fat	Less than	65g	80g
Sat Fat	Less than	20g	25g
Cholesterol	Less than	300mg	300mg
Sodium	Less than	2400mg	2400mg
Total Carbohydrate		300g	375g
Dietary Fiber		25g	30g

You notice that Brand 1 has more calories per serving (180 compared to 150), more saturated fat (4 grams compared to

1 gram), and more sodium (670 milligrams compared to 320). It also has less of the filling nutrients protein (8 grams versus 12 grams) and fiber (4 grams versus 7 grams) than Brand 2. In this case, Brand 2 seems like a better choice.

The more you practice, the easier it gets, and the less time it takes. At a glance, you'll be able to decide what to choose. This is a great trick not only at the supermarket, as in the above example, but when deciding what to order at a restaurant. Who knew, for example, that the grilled chicken salad is higher in calories than a small burger, or that you'd be better off ordering beef with broccoli instead of eggplant with tofu?

Exercise: Well Worth It

If you're already active, good for you! It's a great habit that is helping you stay healthy and energized through this process.

If you're not exercising yet, you might as well start now, as long as you have your doctor's permission. Exercise has all kinds of benefits:

- It burns calories to help you lose weight and maintain weight loss.

- It makes you happier and more confident.

- It reduces stress.

- It tones your muscles.

- It gives you more energy.

- It lowers risk for all kinds of diseases from diabetes and heart disease to osteoporosis and Alzheimer's disease.

Getting Started

The first goal is to get started. First, get your doctor's permission to exercise, and find out whether you have any restrictions on the activities you can do.

Gather what you need, such as comfortable pants and a top, sturdy walking or cross-training shoes, a water bottle, and a good playlist if you're into music. Decide where you're going to work out and what you're going to do. It may be the gym, a local park, or your own home. You could:

- Walk indoors or outdoors

- Lift a few weights

- Try cardio machines such as the elliptical machine or stationary bicycle

- Take a group fitness class, such as boot camp, Zumba, Pilates, or yoga

- Follow a workout video, such as DVD that you buy or borrow from the library, or a video posted on You-Tube

- Grab a buddy or a few for tennis, basketball, Follow the Leader, or beach volleyball

Then hit it!

Whatever you can manage is enough, even if it's only 5 minutes at a slow pace on the treadmill or up and down your driveway, or just making it through the warm-up of an exercise video. The first time out is the hardest. Your body isn't used to it. Plus, your mind may tell you you're bored or tired.

Don't let the soreness, boredom, uncertainty, or fatigue stop you from coming out for your second, third, and fourth tries!

How Much, and What Kind?

Eventually, you can build up your activity to aim to hit national recommendations. These include:

- 75 minutes per week of vigorous activity, such as jogging, singles tennis, or hard cycling OR

- 150 minutes per week of moderate activity, such as brisk walking, dancing, cycling, or swimming

- PLUS

- Strength training each muscle group two times per week.

Strength Training: Not the Same as Body Building

No, lifting weights won't bulk you up. It slims you down. Building strength and increasing your lean muscle mass actually helps you lose weight because it increases your metabolism. Every pound of muscle burns an extra few calories per day compared to a pound of fat. You get the metabolism-boosting benefits even while you're at rest.

Beyond that, building your strength helps you look good, not to mention feel good. You look more toned when you have muscle mass. It sure feels nice to walk around feeling strong and toned. On the inside, know that your muscles are improving your glucose (blood sugar) control!

You can work on your strength in all kinds of ways:

- Use dumbbells, barbells, and the traditional machines at the gym.

- Use a kettlebell and medicine ball.

- Use cables, pulleys, and heavy bands.

- Use your own body weight – think push-ups, sit-ups, planks, squats, dips, and pull-ups, to name a few.

- Improve your home: think shoveling and digging in the yard, and carrying furniture.

Chore or Privilege?

Exercise can be very hard at first. It's physically and mentally challenging. The only good thing about it may be when it's over. That's okay. Feel good about getting it done, and remember that good feeling so it can motivate you to get going next time.

Know that it gets easier over time. Your body will adapt to the exercise, so you start feeling stronger and more energized instead of tired when you work out. Your mind will get used to the exercise, too, and you may find that you think more clearly on days when you work out than on days when you don't.

Finally, do everything you can to make exercise easier. That's not laziness. That's common sense. The easier exercise is, the more likely you are to do it, and to do more of it. You'll still get all the benefits.

First, find activities you enjoy.

- Is walking too boring? Try a Zumba or kickboxing class where you never know what move is coming next, but you know it'll be fun.

- Can't handle the pounding of running? Try spinning or cycling classes, where the teacher talks you through it and you get the heart-pounding, sweat-dripping workout of your life.

- Love to talk? Join a walking group where the conversation lasts for miles, and may not even stop until you finish stretching over coffee and fruit.

Here are some ways to make exercise easier:

- **Work out with friends, or make new workout friends**. You might as well double up workout time with social hour.

- **Exercise when you like to.** Some people like to rev up during the morning hours, others like to use a workout to release stress at the end of the day. Other like a nice shake-out at lunch to break up a long day.

- **Choose a convenient location.** Hit the gym or work up a sweat in the park on the way to or from work, or get your burn on at home. Save time by working out at a location that's not far out of your way.

- **Take care of yourself to give yourself more energy for your workout.** Get plenty of sleep, drink water throughout the day to stay hydrated, and, of course, eat healthy foods.

What do exercise and sugar have in common? The more you get, the more you depend on it, and the more you want!

YOUR CHALLENGE

Your challenge this month is to exercise at least 12 times. That is enough to get you used to moving and grooving, but it leaves you plenty of days to rest and to take care of anything else that comes up during what would have been your exercise time.

You might want to log your activity this month. It'll help you keep track of the number of days you work out, and it will keep you motivated. When you hit your 12 days, you can look at your log and be proud!

THE MEAL PLAN

Meal 1

Meal	Menu
Breakfast	Bagel sandwich: ✓ 1 whole wheat mini bagel ✓ 2 tablespoons non-fat cream cheese ✓ ½ cup canned salmon
Lunch	¼ recipe of sweet potato salad: ✓ 1 pound cooked sweet potatoes ✓ 4 hard-boiled eggs ✓ ¼ cup dill or sugar free sweet pickles, diced ✓ 1 cup non-fat Greek yogurt ✓ 1 teaspoon Dijon mustard ✓ ½ cup celery, diced ✓ ½ cup green or red onion, diced Place on a bed of lettuce or spinach leaves mixed with 1 ounce roasted nuts such as walnuts or sliced almonds. 1 cup strawberries.
Dinner	Burger night. 4 ounces chicken, soy, or turkey burger Lettuce leaves, tomato slices, and onion slices as desired Grilled mushrooms and onions, if wanted Low-calorie condiments such as mustard, sugar-free relish, and pickles ½ reduced calorie, high fiber hamburger bun Baked zucchini fries with 2 teaspoons olive oil 1 ounce dark chocolate

Meal 2

Meal	Menu
Breakfast	¼ recipe cheesy spinach and sweet potato make-ahead breakfast frittata with: ✓ 1 10-ounce package of frozen spinach ✓ 3 eggs ✓ 1 pound cooked shredded sweet potatoes ✓ 1 cup shredded cheese ✓ 1 tablespoon chicken bouillon powder or soup base
Lunch	Pita sandwich with hummus 1 small whole-grain pita, cut in half and spread with ¼ cup hummus, and stuffed with Cooked or raw vegetables of your choice, such as sprouts, lettuce, tomatoes, roasted zucchini, roasted peppers, and roasted eggplant. (optional) 3 ounces grilled chicken breast or ½ cup garbanzo beans. 1 cup grapes
Dinner	3 ounces broiled salmon with teriyaki sauce, fresh grated ginger, fresh grated garlic, and chopped green onions 1 cup steamed vegetable of your choice ½ cup cooked brown rice, whole grain couscous, quinoa, or other whole grain of choice

Chapter 6

The Scale and Helpful Tools

BY MONTH 3, you've got the hang of the balloon. You're eating healthy, getting in a little exercise, and hopefully losing weight and feeling good!

It's time to learn a little bit about some of the tools that can help you be successful. Let's learn about weigh-ins and then we'll talk about some of the help you can get when you're trying to cook healthy.

Take advantage of these tools and tricks, and your journey will be a lot easier!

All about Weigh-Ins

Weight loss is at the heart of this journey. Do you know how to track your weight? Anyone who's ever tried to lose weight knows that the scale can drive you crazy, but there are some things you can do to make it easier on yourself.

The "Proper" Way to Weigh in

No kidding, there's a "right" and a lot of "wrong" ways to weigh in. Do it wrong, and you're asking for trouble. The scale will bounce up and down unpredictably, and you may get discouraged.

Here are some tips for meaningful weigh-ins:

- Weigh yourself at the same time each day – usually in the morning right when you get up or after you work out.

- Wear light clothing and no shoes, or – better yet – weigh yourself without clothes, right after you take a shower.

- You can weigh yourself every day if you like, but only count the number as "official" once per week. Friday morning is often a good choice because a lot of people tend to eat a lot of calories and sodium over the weekend, so weight goes up by Monday.

The Scale, Plus a Grain of Salt

Take the scale seriously, but not too seriously. It tells the truth over time – that is, over weeks and months, it'll go down if you're losing weight, and up if you're gaining weight.

But day to day, you can expect your weight to fluctuate. There can be days when the scale goes up, even if you're doing everything right. You could be losing weight, but the scale could go up for any of these reasons (or others):

- You ate a lot of sodium yesterday and your body is retaining water.

- Your hormones are out of whack: attention ladies at a certain time of the month!

- You got dehydrated and now your body is retaining water to compensate.

- You ate a high-carb meal when you don't normally.

- You weighed in when your stomach was full after eating a big meal.

All of the above situations lead to temporary weight gain, and not a true increase in body fat. The best ways to fight that "gain" are to keep up with your healthy eating plan, stay active, and drink plenty of water.

Stay positive when the scale's driving you crazy. Think of other ways to measure your progress. Think of how much healthier and more energetic you feel. Think how proud you are to be sticking to your diet and exercise plan. Think about the new outfit you bought in a smaller size. Think about your wedding ring fitting, seeing the definition in your calf muscles, and finding out that your cholesterol numbers have dropped since you started losing weight.

The scale can keep you on track, but it's not all about the scale.

Food Shortcuts to Make It Easier

You're busy. You're stressed. You don't have time to cook. There are other things you'd rather do. You know takeout and delivery are not your best options, so what can you do?

You can use some of the many "food shortcuts" you have available to you. Think of these shortcuts as a bridge between cooking from scratch and going out to eat. They give you the best of both worlds: nutritious meals with a minimum of hassle.

When you get a chance, see which of these and other "helper" items your supermarket sells:

- Bagged salad mixes

- Pre-cut fruit and vegetables

- Prepared salads, such as marinated artichoke hearts, three bean salad, and caprese salad, at a salad bar or in the deli or fridge section

- Rotisserie chicken and other ready-to-eat meals, such as eggplant parmesan

- Broth-based, chunky soups

Don't get fooled into thinking "fresh" and "supermarket" mean "healthy." Skip the fried chicken and chicken wings, the pizza, the mayonnaise-laden coleslaw, tuna salad, and other salads, the creamy soups, the ribs, and the oversized sandwiches with too much bread and meat.

No Time for Fresh? No Problem!

You may have days when you simply cannot make it to the grocery store for fresh produce and proteins. What then? Nope, pizza and Chinese take-out are not the answer! Just check your freezer and pantry!

You can always put together a few canned and frozen foods to make your own nutritious meal within minutes. These are a few ideas:

- "Mexican" casserole with fat-free refried beans, canned Mexican-style tomatoes, canned eggs, salsa, and brown rice
- Stir fry with a frozen stir fry veggie mix or frozen veggies of your choice, plus
- A veggie burger served with heated frozen broccoli spears and pureed frozen winter squash seasoned (optional) with salt and pepper
- Tuna or salmon and spinach soup with canned tuna or salmon, fresh or frozen spinach, low-sodium chicken or vegetable broth, and mixed frozen vegetables
- Canned mackerel with canned corn, frozen mixed veggies, and Asian style seasonings
- A frozen whole grain waffle spread with peanut butter and topped with frozen blueberries or other no sugar added frozen fruit

Stock your freezer and pantry and be creative, and you can always have good meals within minutes.

Cook Once Now for Several Meals Later

Preparing food on the weekend is one the most time-tested strategies for many successful long-term losers. It's a life-saver if you're crunched for time. Spend an hour or so in the kitchen once a week, and you can have healthy meals and snacks ready all week long.

Preparing batches of food ahead of time is also helpful if you're on a serious budget. You may simply not be able to shell out the money for pre-cut veggies, prepared salads, and ready-to-eat meal components like pre-cooked chicken breast strips.

When you cook big batches, you have the added cost savings from being able to buy in bulk. You can take advantage of sales on seasonal produce and family packs of chicken and fish. If you don't use up these ingredients quickly enough, you can cook and freeze them so they're ready to add to a meal any time you need them.

What should you cook? You might want to make one or two big batches of a main course. Divide your dish into meal-sized portions, and refrigerate or freeze the extras. Heat each portion up when you need it.

These are some basic ideas for dishes:

- Chili with beans, either vegetarian or with extra lean ground turkey

- Soup, such as vegetable and chicken or beef, or bean, pea, or lentil soup with vegetables

- Chicken, tofu, or fish cooked with vegetables

- Stew with chicken or lean beef and vegetables

- Spinach lasagna with low-fat ricotta, using eggplant or zucchini slices instead of pasta

- Frittatas with eggs, your choice of vegetables, and (optional) grated sweet potatoes or winter squash

- Breakfast sandwiches with cooked eggs and low-fat cheese on whole-grain mini bagels

In addition to cooking, you might want to get some snacks ready. Peel, wash, and cut carrots and cucumbers. You can also prepare sliced red peppers, celery sticks, and broccoli and cauliflower florets to eat whenever you need a filling, low-calorie snack. Wash your fruit, too, so it's more readily available than chips, cookies, and crackers. Finally, you can hard-boil eggs for a grab-and-go protein.

Packaged and Processed: Go or No?

What about frozen and dried meals and canned foods? There are all kinds of packaged meals that you just need to heat and eat, or maybe add an ingredient like chicken to make it a complete meal. They can be awfully tempting. Are they worth your while? They can be, if you're careful!

A lot of frozen, canned, and dried meals are pretty bad. They can be high in calories, not to mention sodium, unhealthy fats, sugars, and refined starch.

These are examples of some of the ones that are often pretty bad:

- Pot pie

- Chicken noodle soup. It's not too high in calories, but each can has more sodium than you need in a day, and very little protein and other nutrients.

- Canned or frozen pasta, such as spaghetti in meat sauce, ravioli, and lasagna

- Standard frozen meals with red meat or fried chicken or fish, pasta or rice, and gravy or cheesy or creamy sauce

- Frozen sandwiches and sandwich pockets, and oversized burritos

- Frozen pizza, especially with pepperoni and sausage

- Breakfasts with sausage, bacon, croissants, biscuits, and pancakes

- Toaster pastries and strudels

- French fries, hash browns, and other fried potatoes

- Canned baked beans, chili con carne, and beef stew

But there's no doubt frozen, canned, and dried meals and meals helpers can give you a lift! Just like you do with other foods, look for choices with a lot of nutrients, and keep your own portion to a small, calorie-controlled amount.

When choosing meals, check calories and portion sizes. Also think about the healthy foods that you're already familiar with.

Here are some more strategies for choosing meals:

- **Frozen breakfasts:** look for egg whites and egg white omelets and scrambles with vegetables, whole-grain English muffins, wraps, or pancakes, turkey bacon and sausage, and low-fat cheese.

- **Frozen entrees:** Look low-fat, reduced-calorie meals with a lean protein such as chicken, fish, shrimp, or tofu, sweet potatoes or whole grain such as whole wheat pasta or brown rice, and steamed vegetables.

- **Canned meals:** Get in the protein and fiber, and look for low-fat options without much sugar. Low-fat, low-sodium turkey chili with beans is a good foundation for a meal.

Keep Planning for Success

Your long-term success depends on healthy food choices. Healthy food choices largely depend on planning ahead so you are not caught without healthy choices, and you do not get so hungry that you overeat. These are some more quick tips for fitting healthy meals into your life so you can keep losing weight when the balloon comes out.

Breakfast

Breakfast can be a rushed meal. You can make it easier on yourself by planning ahead. Know what you'll make, and do what you can the night before. You can make overnight oatmeal, store breakfast sandwiches and wraps in the fridge or freezer, and cut up fruit ahead of time.

You can also help yourself out by having quick options on hand so you can grab them as you're running out of the house in the morning.

Each of these quick breakfast ideas has only 250 to 350 calories, but plenty of nutrients:.

- Whole-grain English muffin with 2 tablespoons of almond butter and ½ cup sliced strawberries.

- 2 hard-boiled eggs with 1 ounce whole grain crackers and 1 tangerine.

- 1 packet instant oatmeal made with skim milk plus ½ ounce pecans or other nuts and 1 cup blueberries.

- 1 cup plain Greek yogurt with 1 chopped medium apple, ½ ounce walnuts, and cinnamon.

- 1 egg scrambled with 1 ounce of low-fat cheese and 2 cups spinach leaves, served in a small high-fiber whole grain tortilla.

If you cannot make your own breakfast, you can pick up a healthy bite to eat from a coffee shop or drive-through. Oatmeal, yogurt, fresh whole fruit and fruit salads, and egg whites are healthy choices that are becoming more common. Remember not to waste your good intentions by blowing your daily calories and sugar on a sweetened coffee drink!

Making Lunch

Compared to fast food, packing your own lunch can pack a nutrient punch and save you calories and fat, not to mention money. Make it!

These are some ideas for making most of your lunch ahead of time, so you do not need to worry about it in the morning as you're rushing around getting ready for the day.

- Pack a salad in a large container and some dressing in a smaller one. Pour the dressing on just when you're ready to eat lunch. Or, just buy single-serve dressing packets or store a bottle of dressing at work.

- Early in the week or on Sunday, cut enough vegetables for the week's lunches. You can have radishes, carrots, celery, and other hardy vegetables to take as crunchy snacks in your lunch.

- Prepare some proteins like hard-boiled eggs, roasted chicken breast, and low-fat tuna salad at the beginning of the week so it's ready to go into your lunch bag when you need it. Yogurt and string cheese are also easy choices, since they're pre-portioned and ready to eat.

- Put leftovers in airtight containers when you finish dinner, and take them with you for lunch the next day.

- Keep healthy snack foods in your pantry in single-serving packets. You can purchase them in single-serving packets, or make your own by dividing up big bags or boxes into smaller portions. Air-popped popcorn, nuts, peanuts, and unsweetened whole grain cereal are all nutritious and non-perishable.

Try to get 1 to 2 servings of vegetables, some protein, and some fruit and/or a healthy starch like a whole grain at lunch. Healthy fats can also slip in there.

These are some examples of lunches that are 300 to 400 calories:.

- A peanut butter and banana sandwich using two slices of whole-wheat bread, plus a cup of grape tomatoes.

- A Greek salad with lettuce, 1 ounce of feta cheese, grape tomatoes, cucumbers, olives, herbs, and 2 tablespoons of light Greek dressing or vinaigrette, plus 1 brown rice cake, plus 1 large apple.

- Leftover chicken breast with a cup of steamed broccoli and a half-cup of cooked brown rice, plus 1 ounce of almonds and a tangerine.

- Plain non-fat Greek yogurt, one ounce of lightly sweetened or unsweetened whole-grain cereal (like bran flakes or shredded wheat), and one cup of berries, plus ½ ounce nuts such as pecans, walnuts, or cashews.

- 1 can (2 cups) of low-sodium chicken vegetable soup with 1 cheese stick (string cheese) melted in, plus 1 cup carrot sticks.

Even with your careful planning, there may be times when you just don't have time to make your own brown -bag lunch. Luckily, fast food is not all bad, and it can be a good choice when you need it. Just choose something sensible. Think grilled chicken rather than a burger or crispy chicken, a salad instead of a wrap or sub sandwich, steamed veggies or carrot sticks instead of fried rice or French fries, and apple slices or yogurt instead of cookies. You'll find mMore tips are in the earlier discussion of fast food in in Chapter 8Month 5..

Dinner

At the end of a long day, you can be tired. You may be short on time if you get home late, have chores to do, and try to catch up with your family. On days like this, dinner can be a mess, but it does not need to be.

Do your best to prepare ahead of time, such as cooking big batches on weekends and doing prep work like cutting veggies and cooking chicken early. Do not forget to take advantage of aids such as frozen and pre-cut veggies and ready-to-eat dishes from the grocery store.

Again, base your meal on vegetables and lean protein, with some high-fiber whole grains or starchy vegetables, too. These are some dinner ideas that are quick to make and add up to 300 or 400 calories:.

- Rotisserie chicken, plus ¼ baked acorn squash, plus a salad with mixed greens and other raw vegetables and 2 tablespoons of light dressing, plus an orange.

- Roasted bell pepper stuffed with lean ground turkey mixed with chunky tomato sauce and topped with parmesan cheese, plus 1 cup steamed Brussels sprouts.

- Fish casserole with white fish, , plus ½ cup fat-free frozen yogurt for dessert.

- Frittata with egg whites, cottage cheese, chopped frozen broccoli and spinach, and seasoning, plus fruit salad and 2 tablespoons whipped topping (optional) for dessert.

- Chicken stew with bell peppers, tomatoes, and zucchini, plus 1 slice whole-grain bread.

- Taco salad with lettuce, diced tomatoes, diced onions, ½ cup fat-free refried beans, 1 ounce shredded cheese, 1 ounce avocado, and ½ cup Greek yogurt.

You can always get part of your meal from a restaurant or the prepared foods section of a supermarket, and pair it with healthy fixings that you have on hand. For example, pick up some all-natural roasted chicken breast and aged parmesan at the deli, dice them, and mix them with a bag of salad for a hearty, healthy meal.

YOUR CHALLENGE

The nutrition label is one of your most powerful weapons in the weight loss battle, but it takes a while to get comfortable reading it. Your challenge is to practice using nutrition labels.

When you are at the grocery store this week, try to use the nutrition label to find out the calories per serving of at least 5 different packaged foods. If that becomes easy for you, go a step further and look for some other information. You could check for:

- **Trans fat:** you should not eat any foods with trans fats!

- **Added sugars in the list of ingredients.** You may be surprised at how many foods have sugar in them. Don't forget to check for sugars like (high fructose) corn syrup, dextrose, honey, dehydrated cane juice, and dextrose.

- **Fiber.** Your goal is at least 20 to 25 grams per day.

THE MEAL PLAN

Meal 1

Meal	Menu
Breakfast	Cottage cheese oatmeal pancakes made with: ✓ ½ cup cottage cheese. ✓ ½ cup oats. ✓ 1 egg. ✓ 1 teaspoon baking powder. ✓ 1 teaspoon cinnamon (optional). ✓ ¼ teaspoon salt. ✓ 2 tablespoons milk or almond milk. ✓ 2 tablespoons chopped pecans or other nuts. ✓ 1 cup blueberries.
Lunch	Greek salad with pita chips. ✓ 2 to 4 cups Romaine lettuce. ✓ 2 tablespoons pitted Kalamata olives (or canned sliced black or green olives). ✓ (optional) ½ cup artichoke hearts. ✓ 1 large tomato, chopped. ✓ ½ cucumber, chopped. ✓ 1/4 cup red onion, diced. ✓ ¼ cup feta cheese. ✓ Lemon juice. ✓ Fresh or dried oregano. ✓ 1 tablespoon olive oil. ✓ ½ medium whole grain pita, toasted and broken into "chips."
Dinner	2 stuffed bell peppers, made with hollowed already-cooked bell peppers and stuffed with: ✓ ½ cup pureed cooked eggplant. ✓ 3 ounces lean ground turkey or crushed veggie burger. ✓ ½ cup Italian style stewed canned tomatoes. ✓ ¼ cup parmesan cheese. 1 cup cut cantaloupe or 1 large orange.

121

Meal 2

Meal	Menu
Breakfast	Southwest egg or tofu scramble: ✓ 2 eggs or ½ cup firm tofu. ✓ ½ cup fresh or frozen corn. ✓ 1 cup cut bell peppers, onions, and tomatoes. ✓ ½ cup canned low-sodium black beans. ✓ 1 teaspoon olive oil for frying. ✓ ¼ cup guacamole or avocado. ✓ ¼ cup salsa.
Lunch	¼ recipe of chicken mushroom vegetable stew: ✓ 2 cups cooked skinless chicken breast. ✓ 2 cloves garlic. ✓ 2 tablespoons olive oil. ✓ 2 cups low-sodium chicken broth. ✓ 2 carrots, 2 stalks celery, and 1 onion, all sliced. ✓ 2 cups sliced fresh mushrooms. ✓ 2 cups cut vegetables such as broccoli, zucchini, tomatoes, or okra. ✓ 2 cups fresh spinach or kale. ✓ 1 cup frozen peas. ✓ 1 cup cubed cooked potatoes. ✓ 1 cup cut cantaloupe or 1 medium apple.
Dinner	4 ounces tilapia or other white fish, broiled with lemon or lime juice and capers (optional). ¼ recipe Asian broccoli salad: ✓ 2 cups broccoli florets. ✓ 1 cup diced red pepper. ✓ 1 cup sliced celery. ✓ 1 tablespoon diced peeled ginger. ✓ 1 cup mandarin orange or tangerine wedges. ✓ 1 tablespoon sesame oil. ✓ 1 teaspoon red pepper flakes. ✓ ¼ cup rice wine vinegar. ✓ ¼ cup low-sodium soy sauce. ✓ ½ teaspoon garlic powder. ✓ Salt, pepper, and low-calorie sweetener to taste.

Chapter 7

Bumps in the Road

THE GASTRIC BALLOON helps, but life still throw challenges at you. What are some of the bumps you can expect, and how will you get over them?

Some of the challenges you'll face are predictable. Getting ready for them can help make it easier for you to surge past them when they do come up.

Some of the common ones that you can get ready for are hitting a plateau in your weight loss, eating when you're not hungry, and hitting the wall with your exercise program.

When the Scale Gets Stubborn: The Dreaded Plateau

A plateau or stall is the name for when you stop losing weight even when you're trying to. It can last for a few days to a few weeks or even longer. It's frustrating. It's infuriating. And it often seems unfair.

A plateau can happen for a lot of reasons. If you've been losing weight steadily for a while, your body may just be ready for a break. This is especially true if you lost a lot of weight within a short period of time. So, you might stop losing weight for a little while, even if you're still sticking to your meal plan and exercise program.

Sometimes, a plateau can happen because you've fallen off the bandwagon. This can even happen without you realizing it. For example, if you stop measuring and logging your food, you could accidentally start eating a little more here and there without meaning to. Those extra bites and calories can add up and cut into your weight loss.

Break through Your Plateau!

There are a few rules for breaking through plateaus can coming out on the other side stronger, healthier, and lighter.

Rule 1: Don't Give Up: It's tempting to throw in the towel. After all, if you're not losing weight when you give up the nachos and ice cream, why *shouldn't* you have them? That's the first line of thinking many people have, but don't let it sway your resolve! Go back to your old habits, and you'll go back your old weight. Guaranteed.

Rule 2: Be Honest: It's hard to accept that a plateau may be fair, but it often is. Your job is to recognize and accept the reason for the plateau. Your plateau may be balancing out some faster-than-expected weight loss in recent weeks (and you probably weren't complaining about that!). Or, your plateau may be the result of sneaky treats and missed workouts. Admit it to yourself if that's the case.

Rule 3: Be Patient and Persistent: Keep doing the right things for weight loss, and you will lose weight. Eat right, exercise, track your food, drink your water, and eat slowly. You will lose weight, whether it takes you a few days or a few weeks to crack that weight barrier.

Rule 4: Give Yourself a Lot of Love: The last thing you may feel like doing during a plateau is loving yourself, but it's a good idea. Get plenty of sleep, reduce stress however you can, and see if you can add in some fun to your days. You just may find that pampering yourself helps the pounds start melting away again.

Rule 5: Shake It Up (Optional): Some people swear by this rule, while others don't think it works. You may be able to break through a plateau by shaking up your routine. The mental boost or physical jolt can sometimes get the scale to move. You could:

- Try eating more meals, but making them smaller

- Try a new kind of workout, like adding strength training if you usually just do cardio

- Drink more fluids if you don't usually drink enough

- Eat a ton of vegetables and cut back on carbs for a few days

"I Just Started Eating…"

Whatever led you to gain weight in the first place is almost sure to rear its ugly head again. Why did you gain weight? Was it:

- Emotional eating?

- Boredom eating?

- Depression eating?

- Making high-calorie choices?

- Social eating?

These situations are going to come up again while you have the gastric balloon and afterward. They are among the biggest challenges you will face. The best thing you can do to protect yourself is to think about them and prepare for them.

Get to the Root

A plateau also may be the result of some erosion in your eating habits, so you need to go back to basics a bit to discover what may be causing your momentum to slow. Now may be a good time to review the "mindful eating" cautions noted in Chapter 4. There are others you may also want to assess.

Making high-calorie choices:

This may have been a major problem before the gastric balloon, especially if you were not an expert on nutrition. Now that you have the balloon system and you have been reading up on and practicing good nutrition, this may not be so much of a problem.

Now you know that sugary foods and beverages, fried and other fatty foods, and starchy foods can pack way more calories than you wanted. You know how to read labels to find lower-calorie foods, and you know to check for protein and fiber because they're filling nutrients.

To reinforce your avoidance of high-calorie choices, you can:

- Opt for vegetables first, since they're generally lowest in calories.

- Add some protein such as fish, fat-free yogurt or cheese, or beans to increase satisfaction and delay the return of hunger.

- Eat when you're hungry but not yet starving, since fatty, sugary, starchy, and high-sodium choices look better when you're starving.

- Get enough sleep, since lack of sleep increases hunger and reduces your ability to resist high-calorie foods.

- Always have low-calorie foods ready to eat. Foods like baby carrots, washed and cut celery and grapes, and air-popped or light popcorn can give you satisfaction without many calories.

- Don't keep high-calorie foods in the house. It's far too easy to down ready-to-eat foods like cookies, chips, and leftover fast food.

- Substitute lower-calorie recipes for higher-calorie ones.

Super Swaps!

There are all kinds of swaps that can help you satisfy cravings for fewer calories. Here are a few ideas:

- "Cauliflower" fried rice for fried rice
- "Zoodles" (zucchini noodles) or spaghetti squash for pasta
- Eggplant or zucchini for lasagna noodles
- Baked chicken and high-fiber crushed cereal instead of fried, battered chicken
- Baked sweet potato or zucchini fries instead of French fries
- Pureed carrots, turnips, or cauliflower instead of mashed potatoes
- Whipped non-fat cream cheese with pumpkin, cinnamon, egg white, and low-calorie sweetener instead of full-fat, full-sugar cheesecake
- Cauliflower and low-fat cottage cheese and cheddar instead of macaroni and cheese

Again, logging is a tool that can help you, once you start to realize how quickly high-calorie foods add up, and how little satisfaction they give, compared with healthy and lower-calorie foods.

Social Eating

If you're hanging with the wrong crowd, your waistline could show the effects. People tend to eat like their friends and family. You know how it goes: you order what everyone else does so you don't stand out, or you don't know what the healthy choices are to order at a restaurant, or you feel obligated to clean your plate multiple times when you're someone's dinner guest.

Getting over unhealthy social eating is a challenge because it involves other people, but you can do it. The first skill you need is the one you've been practicing for months now: recognizing healthy foods and portions. Whether you're at a restaurant or a friend's house, you know to look for veggies, lean proteins, and healthy carbs. You also know to pile on the veggies, and minimize the refined starches and sugars.

The other skill you need is the ability to say, "No, thank you." It's not easy, but you can do it. It may take a little practice. You can keep it to a simple, "No, thank you," or you can add a little explanation if you like. "No, thank you; I'm not hungry anymore." "No, thank you, I don't want any dessert." "No, thank you, my doctor told me not to eat more than a couple bites of white pasta at a time."

Do Something Else – Anything Else!

Find a different outlet instead of eating. Many people think of taking a walk, but when the time comes, they find it easier to hit the fridge. So, your substitute activity doesn't have to be something useful or productive. As long as you don't turn to food, you're coming out on top. You could:

- **Hop on the computer or your smartphone** for some social time by texting or going on discussion forums or social media.

- **Log and plan some meals**, which not only helps you get over the urge to eat, but also helps motivate you to stick to those healthy intentions.

- **Watch TV.** It doesn't exactly burn a lot of calories or stimulate your mind, but it does come with a calorie-free option.

- **Phone a friend.** Just make sure you have a long list of possible friends to call so that if one doesn't answer, you can try calling the next one on the list.

- **Sew, knit, scrapbook, or doodle.** It keeps your hands busy, too, so it's harder to eat!

- **Read** or do crosswords or Sudoku.

- **Fold laundry**, sweep the floor, wash the dishes, or sort the mail.

You see, it doesn't have to involve exercise. But if you do want to get moving instead of eating, go for it! Are you feeling angry? Lift a few weights. Is your mind unfocused? Hit the gym for a group fitness class and just follow the instructions. Do you feel lonely? Take a brisk walk with one or more buddies.

Hitting the Wall with Exercise

Staying true to your new healthy diet is difficult. It also is tough to keep up a long-term exercise program. It can be boring. You may be short on time. Maybe you're not seeing results. Everyone has trouble at some point or other keeping up with their exercise routine.

Problem	Strategies
You don't like exercise.	Keep trying new activities until you find one you like. Make it fun by going with a group of friends, going to a group exercise class with a great teacher, or taking up a sport that doesn't seem just like a workout.
You are bored.	Mix up your activities so you are not consistently doing the same workout. In a single week, you could cycle, walk, lift weights, hike, do yoga, and take a dance class. Try exercising with a friend to prevent boredom, or download a few favorite songs to listen to.
You're not getting results.	This can suck the motivation right out of you, but results are coming. You're burning calories and improving health whether or not you can detect it. To bump up the results, hire a personal trainer for a few sessions, or throw in a little extra intensity or a few extra minutes a couple of times a week.
You have no time.	Schedule it in, just like you schedule in doctor's appointments and meetings at work. When you think of it as something you will do, and not just something you might do, you can fit it in. Try getting in extra steps at lunchtime, while doing errands, and throughout the day by taking short walking breaks.
You are uncomfortable.	Talk to your doctor if your balloon is making you feel uncomfortable while exercising. Try lowering the intensity so it is not as strenuous. If you have pain while exercising, ask an expert such as a trainer for ways you can modify the activity to avoid pain.

The trick is to make it as easy on yourself as possible. That's different from being lazy. Here are some common reasons why people give up, and how you overcome them.

YOUR CHALLENGE

You know how important it is to plan ahead and try to make some meals ahead of time. That's exactly what your challenge is for now. Your goal is to make at least one healthy, multi-serving dish each weekend this month so you can be sure to have some healthy, ready-made meals during the week.

Here are a few ideas for healthy mains and sides.

- Baked oatmeal pancakes with 2 cups oats, ½ cup whole wheat or almond flour, 4 eggs, 1 teaspoon salt, 2 teaspoons baking powder, 2 cups milk, and (optional) 2 packets low-calorie sweetener. Stir, put on cookie sheets, bake, and freeze! Makes enough for 4 breakfasts.

- Cucumber salad with sliced cucumbers, vinegar, peeled diced fresh ginger, diced onion, fresh chopped dill, low-calorie sweetener, and salt and pepper to taste. This lasts for days in the fridge.

- Vegetarian chili with kidney, pinto, garbanzo, and/or black beans, canned tomatoes, diced celery, bell peppers, and onions, and chili seasoning mixed. Optional: lean ground turkey, sliced mushrooms, and eggplant cubes.

- Eggplant beet dip with pureed eggplant, pureed cooked beets, olive oil, minced garlic, lemon juice, and salt to taste. Eat with raw veggies or spread on whole grain pita or bread for a tasty, healthy dip or spread.

- Turkey meatloaf with 1 lb. lean ground turkey, ½ cup oats or cooked quinoa, ½ cup diced onion, 2 cups kale or spinach leaves, 2 eggs, 1 cup grated zucchini, and salt, onion powder, pepper, and ketchup. Bake in a loaf pan, and slice into individual portions before freezing.

THE MEAL PLAN

Meal 1

Meal	Menu
Breakfast	2 egg muffins (1/3 of a 6-muffin recipe) made with: • 6 eggs • ½ cup shredded low-fat cheddar or jack cheese • 1 cup cooked, diced veggies such as zucchini, yellow squash, red and green bell peppers, and broccoli • 3 ounces cooked diced chicken, canned sardines, or vegetarian breakfast sausage • Italian seasoning or fresh or dried rosemary or oregano • Salt and pepper to taste • ½ cup high-fiber cereal in ½ cup unsweetened almond milk
Lunch	2 halves of a small whole grain pita, each spread with 1 tablespoon hummus and stuffed with sprouts, tomatoes, lettuce, and ½ cup of garbanzo beans 1 cup fruit salad with your favorite fruit 1 sugar-free fudge pop
Dinner	Chicken pizzas stuffed on an eggplant base 1 medium eggplant, cooked, halved, hollowed, and stuffed with the following ingredients: • 3 ounces roasted chicken, chopped • ½ cup tomato or marinara sauce • The inside of the eggplant • Cooked mushrooms • ¼ cup shredded low-fat parmesan cheese on top Brown in the broiler.

Meal 2

Meal	Menu
Breakfast	Yogurt parfait: 1 container non-fat plain or no sugar added vanilla Greek yogurt layered with: • 1/3 cup oats mixed with ½ teaspoon cinnamon • ½ ounce (2 tablespoon) chopped walnuts or other nuts • 1 cup fresh or frozen berries – your choice
Lunch	Chicken salad on 3 to 4 cups of romaine lettuce, spinach leaves, or mixed greens: • 4 ounces roasted skinless chicken breast, diced or cut in strips • ½ cup fruit such as pitted cherries, raspberries, tangerine sectors, or peach slices • 1 cup vegetables such as onion slices, grape tomatoes, snow peas, and carrot slices • 2 tablespoons raspberry or balsamic vinaigrette • 1 slice of whole grain bread spread with olive oil, garlic powder, and thyme, toasted, and cut into small crouton-like pieces
Dinner	3 ounces grilled shrimp, 1 tablespoon pine nuts (or chopped peanuts) and ½ cup fresh basil leaves tossed with 1 cup zucchini noodles cooked in chicken broth. 2 graham crackers (the large rectangles) with pumpkin cream cheese: • 2 tablespoons non-fat cream cheese whipped with • 1 tablespoon pumpkin puree • ½ teaspoon cinnamon • Low-calorie sweetener (optional)

Chapter 8

In It for the Long Haul

IT'S ONE THING to follow a strict diet for a few months. Since you got the balloon, you've likely been pretty careful to stick to your meal plans. You may have been able to avoid situations that kept you away from your intended meals.

But sooner or later, you will almost certainly need to get out of your comfort zone. You'll find yourself at a restaurant or a party. You'll find yourself hanging out with or cooking for family and friends. You may need to figure out solutions that let you keep losing weight while you enjoy life. Don't worry – there are solutions!

Restaurants: Let Someone Else Do the Healthy Cooking

While you may prepare most of your meals at home, you'll be eating restaurant-prepared food at some point. Whether it's fast food or a meal from a casual or fine dining restaurant, you can find options that are diet-busting, diet-saving, and everything in between.

The game plan stays the same as it does when you're cooking for yourself. Load up on veggies and fruit and add some lean protein. Then think about a serving of starch from whole grains or starchy veggies. As you're used to doing, skip sugary food and extra fats.

Does that sound like what you've been practicing for months now? It's that simple!

Your Energizing Breakfast

You have plenty of options if you don't get a chance to make yourself breakfast. If you can't find an egg white scramble with vegetables, your best bet may be to look for some fresh fruit and a container of yogurt. These suggestions can help you get a healthy breakfast nearly anywhere.

Look for:	Skip:
✓ Egg whites	Cinnamon rolls and bear claws
✓ Fresh fruit or fruit salads	Donuts, fritters, and other fried foods
✓ Non-fat, plain or no sugar added yogurt	Full-size bagels (especially white) and full-fat cream cheese
✓ Oatmeal	Sugar-sweetened coffee drinks, especially with cream or whipped cream
✓ Cold cereal, especially unsweetened and whole grain	Maple syrup, brown sugar, and other sugary toppings
✓ Ham and turkey bacon and sausage*	Sausage and bacon
✓ Breakfast sandwiches with egg whites on an English muffin	Pancakes and waffles unless whole grain
	Breakfast platters
	Hash browns and other fried foods

*low in calories and high in protein, but may contain cancer-causing nitrates

Fast Food: Fast Nutrition or Fast Calories?

Fast food restaurants have a pretty bad reputation in general, but most have improved their offerings. Almost all chains now offer a few healthy choices on their menus. Furthermore, many are willing to customize your order for you. For example, you may be able to ask for:

- The bun on the side, or your burrito in a bowl.

- A side of steamed vegetables instead of rice.

- Thin crust or whole-wheat crust and no cheese on your pizza.

- Dressings on the side.

These suggestions can help you get a healthy lunch at nearly any kind of fast food joint.

Look for:	Skip:
Burger Joints	
• Kids'-sized burgers, especially without the bun • Side salads • Baby carrots, yogurt, and fruit for sides • Veggie burger patties and grilled chicken	• French fries, onion rings, zucchini sticks, and other fried sides • Double or triple sized burgers • Shakes, floats, and soft drinks
Sandwiches	
• Whole grain bread or wraps • Your sandwich in a salad • Grilled chicken, all-natural turkey and ham • Extra vegetables • Low-carb wraps • Lettuce wraps	• Already dressed salads • Fatty cold cuts such as pepperoni, salami, and bologna • Double meat and cheese • Mayonnaise-based tuna salad • Oversized sub rolls, bagels, and baguettes. • Bacon
Mexican	
• Small tacos • Salads without tortilla chips or tostada shells • Fajitas without tortillas • Black beans • Salsa, tomatoes, and shredded lettuce	• Loaded burritos • Quesadillas • Tostadas • Nachos and tortilla chips • Sour cream • Options with fried dough, such as chimichangas and churros

Look for:	Skip:
Asian	
• Steamed vegetables • Stir fry with vegetables and chicken, shrimp, or fish	• Fried rice and chow mein • Breaded chicken, fish, and shrimp • Sweet and sour dishes • Pot-stickers and fried dumplings • Egg rolls and spring rolls
Cafes	
• Broth-based soups, such as chicken noodle, minestrone, and vegetable beef • Salads with dressing on the side • Whole-grain bread	• Sugar-sweetened coffee and other drinks • Cream soups • White bread, bagels, and rolls • Salad toppings such as bacon, chow mein noodles, and croutons
Pizza	
• Thin, whole-wheat crust • Little or no cheese • Vegetable toppings: mushrooms, peppers, tomatoes, spinach, and onions • Extra sauce • Chicken breast and anchovies • Side salads with dressing on the side	• Thick-crust and deep-dish • Stuffed crust • Pepperoni, sausage, and meat lover's pizza • Double cheese • More than one slice • Breadsticks, cheese sticks, and cinnamon sticks • Creamy dipping sauces such as ranch

Still not convinced you can eat healthy at fast food joints? Choose one of the breakfasts, and two of the lunches/dinners from the following list, and you'll come in under 1,200 calories and get some good nutrients, too. Top off your meal with a low-calorie drink, and you won't be doing too badly!

Breakfasts

- McDonald's Egg White Delight or Egg McMuffin and Cuties (tangerines).

- McDonald's Fruit n' Yogurt Parfait and Apple Slices.

- McDonald's Fruit & Maple Oatmeal and Apple Slices.

- Burger King Fruit Topped Maple Flavored Oatmeal.

- Burger King Maple Flavored Oatmeal with Fat-Free Milk.

- Wendy's Steel Cut Oatmeal without brown sugar.

- Taco Bell Egg and Cheese Egg and Cheese A.M. Grilled Taco.

- Subway 6" Egg White and Cheese or Egg White and Cheese with Ham, plus low-fat milk.

- Starbucks Classic Whole-Grain with Nut Medley Topping and Dried Fruit.

- Starbucks Blueberry Oatmeal with Fruit, Nut, and Seed Medley Topping

- Starbucks Reduced Fat Turkey Bacon Breakfast Sandwich or Spinach & Feta Breakfast Wrap with Seasonal Harvest Fruit Blend.

- Starbucks Greek Yogurt Parfait.

- Chick-Fil-A Chicken, Egg, and Cheese Bagel plus a Small Fruit Cup (eat only half the bagel).

- Chick-Fil-A Greek Yogurt Parfait plus a Large Fruit Cup.

Lunches/Dinners

- McDonald's Artisan Grilled Chicken Sandwich plus a Side Salad with Low-Fat Balsamic Vinaigrette or Low-Fat Italian Dressing and Apple Slices.

- McDonald's Premium Southwest Salad with Grilled Chicken plus Cuties (clementines).

- McDonald's Hamburger plus a Side Salad with Low-Fat Balsamic Vinaigrette or Low-Fat Italian Dressing plus Go-Gurt.

- Burger King Flame-Grilled Chicken Burger, Tendergrill Chicken Sandwich, or Veggie Burger no mayo, plus a Garden Side Salad, no dressing or Light Vinaigrette.

- Burger King Garden Grilled Chicken Salad.

- Wendy's Jr. Hamburger plus Apple Slices and a Garden Side Salad with Light Spicy Asian Vinaigrette and no croutons.

- Wendy's Grilled Chicken Wrap with lettuce and tomato plus a Garden Side Salad with Light Spicy Asian Vinaigrette and no croutons.

- Wendy's Baked Potato with Broccoli (skip the cheese) and a Small Rich & Meaty Chili.

- Wendy's Half Size Asian Cashew Chicken Salad or Power Mediterranean Salad plus a Small Rich & Meaty Chili.

- Taco Bell Cantina Power Bowl Fresco Style.

- Taco Bell Chicken or Steak Soft Taco plus Pintos n'Cheese.

- Taco Bell Bean or Chicken Burrito, Fresco Style.

- Subway sandwiches from 6 grams of fat or less menu on 9-Grain Wheat or Multigrain Flatbread with tons of vegetables and mustard or any low-fat dressing.

- Subway Beef Chili.

- Subway Black Bean, Chicken and Wild Rice, or any other soup with 200 or fewer calories, plus Apple Slices.

- Subway Veggie Delite Salad or any 6 grams of fat or less salad, or Double Chicken Chopped, Rotisserie-Style Chicken, or Turkey Salad with fat-free Italian dressing.

- Starbucks Zesty Chicken & Black Bean Salad Bowl or Hearty Veggie & Brown Rice Salad Bowl.

- Starbucks Bistro Boxes.

- Pizza Hut 4 Traditional (not breaded) Wings with a Marinara Dipping Cup plus a Garden Salad with Light Italian Vinaigrette Salad Dressing.

- Pizza Hut 2 slices Veggie Lover's Small Hand-Tossed plus a Garden Salad with Light Italian Vinaigrette Salad Dressing.

- KFC Kentucky Grilled Breast plus Green Beans plus Whole Kernel Corn.

- KFC 2 Kentucky Grilled Thighs plus a House or Caesar Side Salad, no croutons, with Light Italian or Fat Free Ranch Dressing.

- Chipotle Salad Bowl with lettuce, your choice of chicken, steak, barbacoa, fajitas, or sofritas, Fresh Tomato Salsa, and Black or Pinto Beans.

- Chick-Fil-A Grilled Market Salad.

- Chick-Fil-A Grilled Chicken Sandwich with a Fruit Cup.

- Chick-Fil-A Medium Hearty Breast of Chicken Soup with a Large Superfood Side.

- Chick-Fil-A Large Hearty Breast of Chicken Soup with Side Salad.

Low-Calorie Beverages

- Water

- Decaffeinated coffee

- Hot tea

- Unsweetened ice tea

Sit-Down Restaurants: The Chef Can Work for Your Health!

Fast food restaurants may have the worst reputation, but sit-down restaurants can be just as bad or even worse. A meal from a sit-down restaurant can end up being bigger and less healthy than a meal from a fast food restaurant.

Your game plan here is to keep it simple and small. Pass up the bread basket and most of the appetizers. Instead, go for salads or non-creamy soups for your starters. When ordering your main course, avoid fatty meats and look for a lean protein such as chicken or fish. Choose one that is not breaded or fried, and has no creamy or cheesy sauce. Get vegetables for a side, pass up dessert, and you've got a healthy meal!

These suggestions can help you get a healthy meal nearly anywhere.

Look for:	Skip:
• Shrimp cocktail appetizers • Raw vegetables • Grilled, roasted, braised, stewed, and steamed as cooking methods • Grilled or roasted skinless chicken and fish • Steamed vegetables and fresh fruit • Side salads and entrée salads • Sauces and dressings on the side • Fresh fruit	• Fried appetizers such as fried mozzarella sticks and calamari • Creamy dips, such as blue cheese, artichoke, and spinach • Breadsticks, rolls, chips, and other pre-meal munchies • Salads that are already dressed • Salad toppings such as cold cuts, croutons, cheese, and bacon • Creamy soups • Most pasta dishes* • Creamy and cheesy sauces • Fried, creamed, battered, crispy, au gratin, and breaded as cooking methods • Fatty meats such as ribs and steaks • Starchy sides, such as potatoes, white rice, and pasta • Desserts such as ice cream, cake, and pie

*They can have 4 or more servings of pasta in a single order.

If you don't see something on the menu that fits into your meal plan, you can ask. Many restaurants are happy to cater to you, and here some ways you can get a meal that works for you.

- They may be so kind as to serve you a specially cooked meal, such as some grilled chicken breast or fish with steamed veggies, for example.

- If they don't want to do that, you could ask for something that takes almost no preparation, such as a scoop of tuna or cottage cheese plus some fruit or a side salad.

- You could order the regular meal and eat only the parts you want, such as eating the salad and the chicken without breading, but skipping the bread and fries from a breaded chicken sandwich platter.

Portion size is one of the biggest problems at restaurants. Here's a way you can protect yourself. Stop for a minute after you are served and before you eat. Look at your food, and decide how much you should eat at the meal. Pack the rest up before you take your first bite. You can have the leftovers for your next meal.

Get the Facts

The law is on your side. Since December of 2015, all restaurants with more than 20 locations nationwide have been required to post certain nutritional information on their menus.[11] This includes printed and board menus at the restaurant, as well as menus posted online. The law covers restaurants, bakeries, cafes, coffee shops and all kinds of food service establishments. That's great news for watching your weight!

The required information includes:

---

11   http://www.fda.gov/Food/IngredientsPackagingLabeling/Labeling-Nutrition/ucm217762.htm

- Calories

- Total fat calories and grams

- Saturated fat

- Trans fat

- Cholesterol

- Sodium

- Total carbohydrate grams

- Dietary fiber

- Sugar

- Protein

This is great news! Knowing the calorie and nutrient counts lets you build a meal that fits into your diet – no nasty surprises necessary!

You can check the nutrition information online before you visit the restaurant. Choose a starter, main course, and side that fits within your calorie budget. When you get to the restaurant, you don't need to even look at the menu. Just order your pre-planned meal and relax.

Even if you don't get a chance to check the facts before going to a restaurant, you can find out what you need to know before ordering. Just check the menu! You can also look up most restaurants' information online by going directly to the restaurant's website or by looking it up in your usual food logging app.

By the way, the law requiring calorie counts on menus applies to amusement parks, movie theaters, bowling alleys, and other entertainment venues with at least 20 locations serving similar foods. "Restaurant type" (ready to eat) food sold in grocery stores is also covered by the law.

Blatant Enemies and False Friends: Beware the False Friends

How bad can a restaurant meal be? It can be pretty bad if you make the wrong choices and go overboard on the portions. Consider this meal:

- Coconut shrimp (600 calories)

- Fettuccini Chicken Alfredo (1,200 calories)

- New York Style Cheesecake (700 calories)

- Soft Drink (200 calories)

This single meal adds up to 2,700 calories – more than two days' worth on your balloon meal plan!

Curious about how bad some of the dishes can be? Here are a few shockingly high-calorie items you could order.

- Mushroom Swiss Burger with French Fries: 1,600 calories

- Beef and Bean Burrito: 1,300 calories

- Lasagna or Spaghetti and Meatballs: 1,000 calories

- Chili Cheese Fries: 400 calories

- Hot Fudge Brownie: 1,400 calories

Not all of the "bad" choices are so obvious. Sometimes you think you're doing yourself a favor by choosing a "diet" type or healthy sounding meal, but you end up with a meal that's just as bad as the decadent ones.

- **Bagel and cream cheese.** You might think you're doing a good thing by choosing a bagel instead of a doughnut, but you'll be getting more calories and fat when you opt for a bagel and cream cheese from a bakery. Add in a sweetened coffee, and you could hit over 700 calories before your day really gets going. A better choice is a bowl of oatmeal or some yogurt and fruit.

- **Salads.** The first thing you look for on the menu may be the worst. Dressings can add hundreds of calories to a salad along with the hundreds from cheese, dried fruit, crispy chicken, and bacon. That's before you even count toppings such as chow mein noodles, sesame sticks, and croutons. A salad can have over 1,000 calories. Instead, stick to salads with greens, other vegetables, fresh fruit, lean protein, and dressing on the side.

- **Wraps.** That innocent looking thin wrap can have more calories and carbs than the sub roll or sliced bread you're avoiding. The wrap itself can have 300 or more calories, with the entire sandwich delivering nearly 1,000 if you go all out on meat, cheese, and sauces. Go for a lettuce wrap or get your salad in a bowl.

- **Soup and sandwich.** A creamy or cheesy soup with croutons together with a hearty sandwich with meat, cheese, and mayo or a creamy sauce can mean you get over 1,000 calories in what you thought was a light lunch. Go for a broth-based soup with a salad instead.

- **Smoothies.** They can be packed with nutritious fruit, but they're also likely to have tons of sugar, both from fruit and from honey or other added sugars. Add in extras like peanut butter, ice cream or frozen yogurt, avocado, and shots of protein or energy blends, and you can be looking at 800 or more calories. Go for water instead, and eat your fruits and veggies as whole foods.

- **Low-fat desserts.** They're usually higher in sugar than regular desserts, and have about as many calories. Go for fresh fruit for a low-fat dessert.

- **Low-carb desserts.** They're usually higher in fat than regular desserts, and have about as many calories. Ask for yogurt instead.

Combining Health with Life

No matter what you are doing in life, you can make it fit into your new healthy lifestyle. You can go out with friends, attend social events and work dinners, and be as involved in your family life as you want while you stay healthy. Here are some things to think about to help you integrate your healthy habits into your life.

Family Meals

You do not need to alienate yourself from your family just because you are eating healthy. Sticking to your special diet can be as simple as taking smaller portions than everyone else in your family.

Another strategy involves avoiding one or two items on the dinner table. For example, you might skip the mashed potatoes when you're serving chicken, mashed potatoes, and green beans. Or, you could have tofu stir fry but skip the white rice.

You can also prepare yourself a similar but separate meal without much effort. If you're making everyone else chicken noodle casserole, for example, you could just set aside your own diced chicken instead of adding it to the casserole with everyone else's portions. Mix it into your salad for your own hearty dinner while everyone else has the casserole.

Buffet style dinners such as taco, burger, pasta, and salad bars are fun ways to get everyone involved and to give yourself healthy options. You can set out the ingredients – even ask your children to help you if possible – and let everyone serve themselves. You can serve:

- **Taco bars:** Taco shells, taco-seasoned ground beef, cooked white fish, and shredded chicken, shredded lettuce, diced tomatoes, shredded cheese, fat-free refried beans, salsa, and guacamole.

- **Burger:** Any kind of burger patty such as ground turkey, veggie, or ground beef, condiments such as relish, mustard, and ketchup, tomato and onion slices, grilled eggplant and zucchini, whole grain buns, cheese slices, and cooked mushrooms.

- **Pasta:** Cooked pasta and spaghetti squash, marinara sauce, meatballs made of ground turkey, parmesan cheese, and cooked vegetables such as cauliflower, broccoli, spinach, and carrots.

- **Salad:** Lettuce and other greens, chopped vegetables such as mushrooms, cucumbers, onion, bell peppers, and tomatoes, sliced hard-boiled eggs, diced chicken breast, tuna, or all-natural turkey breast, shredded cheese, sunflower seeds, nuts, raisins, and tangerine or orange wedges, plus dressings.

These fun dinners let everyone eat what they love while you get to eat healthy, too.

Parties and Get-Togethers – Guaranteed Diet-Friendly

Social events can be tough food-wise. Luckily, you can take charge and make sure there will be at least some foods there you can eat. If you are hosting the party, just make one or more dishes you can enjoy without going over your calories. If you're a guest, be a polite one and bring a dish or two.

These are some great party dishes to serve or bring:

- **Salads.** Start with a base of lettuce, spinach, or mixed greens, and add whatever you like! Sunflower and pumpkin seeds, nuts, diced turkey, tangerine slices, diced pear, red onions, pomegranate seeds, and roasted beets are just a few fun and healthy ingredients. Dress it with a low-fat dressing.

- **Veggies and dip.** Baby carrots, celery sticks, radishes, snow peas, bell pepper strips, and broccoli and cauliflower florets are just the beginning.

- **Dips.** Consider salsa, low-fat bean dip, fat-free Greek yogurt with dill, and hummus as dips you can eat. You can even bring a creamy dip, such as ranch or onion, if you think everyone else will like it, and just stick to the veggies yourself.

- **Fresh fruit.** Cut melon, pineapple, and watermelon, grapes, strawberries, and orange slices are all good party items.

- **Skewers.** Skewers always look fancy at a party. Try combinations such as mozzarella, olive, and cherry tomatoes, grilled shrimp, pineapple, and green pepper, meatball, roasted eggplant, and button mushrooms, and fruit with cubes of cheese.

You may face pressure to eat foods you know you'll regret. Friends and family are excited to share their dishes with you, or they think you'll enjoy the event more if you eat what they offer, or they (unfortunately) may try to sabotage your diet.

Go back to practicing your "No, thanks." "No, thanks. I'm not hungry." "No, thanks. My doctor said I should not eat that." "No, thanks. I cannot eat that." "Not right now, thanks. Maybe later. It looks fantastic!"

Loving Life Beyond Food

The last few chapters have been pretty focused on food, but the purpose is actually the opposite. The reason you have the balloon is to take control of your health, weight, and eating habits. Then, you can focus less on food, and more on life!

You should appreciate the company and conversation. When you're at restaurants, home-made meals with family, and parties with friends, the food is only a small part of the attraction. At amusement parks, you can get caught up in the rides; at the mall, you can shop for the biggest bargains on clothes, not at the food court. Life really does have a lot more to offer than food, and getting control over food can help you see what there is.

You can have a good deal more freedom to enjoy the rest of what life has to offer when you're not focusing on food, when your body is smaller than it was before, and when you have more energy and stamina.

Fun Times Can Be Healthy Times

Wherever you go and whatever you do with family and friends, remember to pack a healthy lunch basket and plenty of water before you go out for the day. That way, you can get involved in whatever activity you're doing without needing to stop to find a healthy lunch.

The Healthy Picnic Basket

You can take a healthy picnic wherever you go. Skip the fried chicken, coleslaw, and chocolate chip cookies, and go for lighter fare that won't weigh you down. Pack your food in an insulated cooler if you're worried about food safety.

- Hard-boiled eggs

- Broccoli slaw or cabbage salad with diced apples, light Asian dressing, and water chestnuts

- Pinwheel sandwiches: use whole wheat flatbread (lavash) or whole grain high-fiber wraps or tortillas. Spread them with a thin layer of fat-free cream cheese or hummus, then add sliced turkey, low-fat cheese, lettuce, and diced tomatoes. Roll the tortilla or lavash, and slice it so you get pinwheel sandwiches.

- Veggie burger patties served on reduced-calorie rolls

- Sweet potato or cauliflower salad with Greek yogurt and dill

- Baby carrots, radishes, and cucumbers with fat-free bean dip, hummus, or roasted eggplant dip

- Brown rice salad with sliced olives, cashews, green onions, olive oil, and sweet fruit such as mangos or pineapples

- Kebabs with mozzarella, cherry tomatoes, cucumbers, and basil

- Peeled or quartered oranges

- Apples

- Cut watermelon

- Bottled water!

If you do get caught without your own healthy snacks or lunch, stay calm. You can do this! Almost every place has some choices that you can work into your diet. Plus, no matter where you are, you get to choose how much you eat. These are some examples of how you can make the best of an imperfect situation and keep enjoying your day out guilt-free.

If You're At:	Skip:	Try:
Amusement and theme parks	Funnel cakes, turkey legs, sweetened beverages, cotton candy, anything deep fried	Corn on the cob, water, pickles, grilled chicken, salads, apples and oranges
Movie theaters	Buttered popcorn, large boxes of candy, nachos, sodas	Bringing your own air-popped popcorn and bottles of water
Mall food courts	Cinnamon rolls and other baked goods such as muffins and brownies, sweetened coffee drinks, pretzels (especially buttered or with cheese or frosting dipping cups), pizza, burgers, chili dogs, and burritos, smoothies	Steamed vegetables and stir fry chicken or beef with vegetables, water, Greek salads or lettuce based salads with grilled chicken and without dressing, a small burger without the bun, thin crust pizza without cheese

YOUR CHALLENGE

Motivation can dip as time passes, but you can learn to motivate yourself for the long term. One great way to do that is to set challenging but achievable goals, and reward yourself when you hit them. Your challenge this month is to set at least three separate goals, each with their own reward.

These are some possible goals:

- Eat at least three servings of vegetables at least five days in a week

- Try a new group fitness class at your gym and go at least three times before you decide whether you like it

- If you normally eat out, bring your lunch to work at least four days in the work week

- Make your breakfast the night before at least four times this week

- Park your car at the far corner of every parking lot you park at this week

These are some possible rewards.

- Call a friend to see a movie with you.

- Buy yourself a new spiralizer, peeler, or anther kitchen gadget that will make healthy cooking more fun or easier.

- Buy that new shirt you've been eyeing for a while and finally fit into.

- Schedule a session with a personal trainer.

THE MEAL PLAN

This meal plan sticks to about 1,200 calories a day and continues to focus on healthy choices. Remember you can always add healthy snacks from if you need more calories. There's a Healthy Snack List in Appendix C.

Meal 1

Meal	Menu
Breakfast	Banana nut oatmeal made with: ✓ ½ cup quick cooking or regular oats ✓ ½ cup unsweetened almond milk ✓ ½ banana. ✓ ½ teaspoon cinnamon ✓ ½ teaspoon vanilla ✓ 2 tablespoons chopped pecans or walnuts
Lunch	1 cup low-sodium, low-fat tomato soup. Grilled cheese: ✓ 2 slices low-calorie, high-fiber bread spread with ✓ 2 teaspoons olive oil ✓ 2 slices ✓ 2 slices tomato ✓ (optional) basil or spinach leaves 1 cup cucumber sticks with ¼ cup Greek yogurt mixed with fresh dill.
Dinner	3 ounces salmon cooked in a pan with 2 teaspoons olive oil and salt and pepper to taste. 1 cup sugar snap peas tossed with ¼ cup thinly sliced green onion, 1 tablespoon vinegar, 1 packet low-calorie sweetener, lime juice, and ¼ teaspoon garlic salt. 2 plums or 1 pear.

Meal 2

Meal	Menu
Breakfast	Breakfast burrito: ✓ 1 small high-fiber wrap ✓ 1 cooked egg ✓ ¼ avocado, sliced ✓ 2 ounces all-natural turkey breast
Lunch	Bulgur salad: ✓ ½ cup cooked bulgur, barley, or farro ✓ ½ cup garbanzo beans ✓ ½ cup artichoke hearts ✓ 1 cup chopped tomato ✓ 2 teaspoons olive oil ✓ Lemon juice, salt, pepper, and parsley to taste 1 apple.
Dinner	¼ recipe of chicken breast, fish, or tofu stewed in pineapple citrus salsa: ✓ 1 lb skinless chicken breast, tilapia, or tofu ✓ 1 grapefruit and 1 orange, each peeled, in sections ✓ 1 cup fresh or frozen pineapple or mango ✓ 1 jalapeno, chopped (optional) ✓ Lime juice ✓ Salt and pepper to taste 1 cup roasted or steamed brussels sprouts ½ cup fat-free frozen yogurt with ½ cup berries

Chapter 9

Looking Ahead

YOU'VE BEEN AT it for a five months now, and hopefully the journey has been pretty exciting. You've learned a lot. You're dropping weight. You're feeling good.

You've spent the past several months focusing on your diet. You may have gained a whole new interest in food, this time from a healthy perspective. With your new knowledge and outlook, you may be interested in improving your diet even more for the maximum benefits in health and weight loss.

Low-Carb, Paleo, Gluten-Free, and Vegetarian: Deserving of the Hype?

You are definitely not alone! Diet plans like low-carb, Paleo, vegetarian, and gluten-free diets are all the rage now. Supporters promise weight loss and better health. Can they deliver? Should you join the millions of other Americans who follow these types of diets?

This is a run-down of some of the most popular current diet fads, and the information you need to decide whether they are for you.

Low-Carb: Does Avoiding Carbs Burn Fat?

Normally, your body get most of its energy from carbohydrates. The premise of low-carb diet is pretty simple: you restrict carbohydrate intake to force your body to burn fat – presumably body fat – for energy.

What You Eat: There are many variations of a low-carb diet. Still, a low-carb diet generally forbids low-nutrient carbohydrates, including:

- Sugar-sweetened beverages, such as soft drinks, sweetened coffee and tea, sports drinks, and fruit drinks

- Sugar-sweetened foods such as candy

- Baked goods such as pies, cookies, and cakes

- Desserts such as ice cream and pudding

- Refined grains, such as white bread, white pasta, and white rice

- Potatoes

- Snack foods such as chips, pretzels, and crackers

- The diet also severely limits more nutritious carb sources:

- Whole grains, such as oatmeal, barley, whole-grain bread and pasta, and brown rice

- Starchy vegetables, such as sweet potatoes, corn, peas, and butternut squash

- Beans, split peas, and lentils

- Fruit

- Yogurt

THE GOOD: A low-carb diet can help you lose weight. You're bound to lose weight if you typically eat high-carb foods like bagels, sandwiches, pasta, rice, burritos, pizza, and desserts, and you cut them out of your diet. If you love carb-free foods like fish, meat, and eggs, you might enjoy this meal plan!

THE BAD: A low-carb diet can be unhealthy. You may replace healthy, high-carb foods like yogurt, oatmeal, and sweet potatoes with high-saturated fat, low-carb foods like bacon, cheese, and butter. That may be bad news for your heart, kidneys, and liver over time.

Speaking of time, a low-carb diet may be hard to follow for a long time. You may eventually crave bread, rice, potatoes, or any other number of carbohydrates. If you bring them back into your diet and feel like you're cheating, you may just give up on your low-carb lifestyle and go back to old eating patterns.

The Bottom Line: A low-carb diet may help you jump-start weight loss or get motivated, but a healthy-carb diet is more sustainable. If you can choose healthy carbs and keep them in small portions, you'll be far better off losing weight and keeping it off.

Paleo: Should You Eat Like a Caveman?

A Paleo diet is supposedly based on an eating pattern that cavemen followed. The premise is that human bodies are not designed for the foods we currently eat, but rather the foods that cavemen ate tens of thousands of years ago. The idea is that cavemen didn't get the chronic diseases such as cancer, heart disease, and osteoporosis that are rampant today.

What You Eat: You can eat what the cavemen presumably ate, although there is some debate on this. A Paleo diet could include:

- Fruits and vegetables

- Plant-based oils, such as olive, flaxseed, and canola

- Nuts and seeds

- Seafood and grass-fed meats

- Eggs

Paleo diets tend to exclude:

- Refined sugar, such as white sugar and foods that contain it

- Processed foods

- Added salt

- Legumes: beans, split peas, lentils, and peanuts[12]

- Potatoes

- Grains, both whole and refined

- Dairy, such as milk, cheese, and yogurt

THE GOOD: A Paleo diet recommends eliminating processed foods, which are often high in calories, blood pressure-raising sodium, artery-clogging trans fats, and added sugars. It also promotes heart-healthy and weight-friendly foods such as nuts, plant-based oils, fruits, vegetables, and seafood.

THE BAD: A Paleo diet excludes many healthy foods. Cutting out dairy can lead to low calcium intake and an increased risk of osteoporosis and risk for bone fractures. Eliminating beans and grains lowers your intake of healthy nutrients such as fiber, potassium, and antioxidants. And there is no evidence that peanuts are unhealthy.

Skeptics of Paleo diets also point out that cavemen did not live very long. They may not have lived long enough to develop chronic diseases that affect humans today. The reason why

---

12   Nutritionists and this book tend to consider peanuts as nuts for nutritional purposes. Botanically and for the purposes of the Paleo diet, they are legumes.

they may not have had heart disease and cancer may have been because they died of other causes – and not because of this diet.

THE BOTTOM LINE: Limiting sugar, salt, and processed foods can only be a good thing. However, if you're going to follow a Paleo-type diet, you might want to include whole grains and legumes in your diet. It will be easier to follow, more enjoyable, more sustainable and probably healthier.

Vegetarian: The Devil Is in the Details

Vegetarian diets have become more mainstream. They promote plant-based foods and limit or exclude animal-based foods. Plant-based diets can be heart-healthy and good for weight loss, and there are tons of meat substitutes that can help you avoid meat without missing it too much.

WHAT YOU EAT: There are many types of vegetarian diets. These are the common ones.

- **Pesco-vegetarian:** excludes meat and poultry.

- **Vegetarian:** excludes meat, poultry, and seafood.

- **Vegan:** excludes all animal-based products, including meat, poultry, seafood, eggs, and dairy products.

THE GOOD: A vegetarian diet encourages healthy foods such as fruits, vegetables, and beans. These choices are filling, high-fiber, and relatively low-calorie: ideal for weight loss. Protein is far less of a problem than most people believe on a vegetarian or even vegan diet.

Plant-based diets also have benefits for the environment. It takes far less energy to produce plant-based foods than meat.

THE BAD: A vegetarian diet is not necessarily healthy by definition. Load up on sugar, starches, and buttery foods, and you're not going to lose more weight or see any health benefits compared to a diet with meat. You still need to choose your foods and watch portions carefully, vegetarian, vegan, or not.

THE BOTTOM LINE: If you're going to go vegetarian, continue to make healthy choices. As you would with any other healthy diet, load up on vegetables, choose healthy fats like avocados, oils, and nuts instead of unhealthy ones like butter, and watch your portion sizes.

As for nutrient consumption, protein is likely not a problem. If you avoid dairy and eggs, you can easily meet your needs using beans, grains, nuts, and soy-based products like tofu. You may need a vitamin B12 supplement if you go vegan, since vitamin B12 is only naturally found in animal products. Also be sure to get enough calcium – typically obtained from dairy products – and iron – whose best sources are meat and other animal foods.

Gluten-Free: Hearsay or Scientifically Backed?

Gluten-free diets have reached epic proportions, and a serious question is, "*why?*" They make perfect sense if you are gluten-sensitive, gluten-intolerant, or have celiac disease. In fact, a gluten-free diet is the only way to handle those conditions.

And for the other millions of Americans who limit gluten? Some think it makes them feel better. Others do it because they think it's healthier. It may be one amazing indication of the great power of marketing from the food industry.

WHAT YOU EAT: A gluten-free diet excludes gluten, which is a protein in wheat, some other grains, and products containing these ingredients. A gluten-free diet excludes:

- Wheat flour and products containing it, such as baked goods

- Wheat bread, pasta, and cereal

- Soy sauce and many other packaged sauces, dressings, and gravies (read the label)

- Beer

- Barley, semolina, graham, spelt, farina, and rye

- Crackers and tortilla chips

- Many processed foods such as deli meats and imitation seafood

You can have:

- Oatmeal, rice, quinoa, sorghum, corn, flax, and buckwheat

- Foods labeled as "gluten-free"

- Soy

THE GOOD: A gluten-free diet can save your life if you're gluten-sensitive. It can also encourage you to eat fewer processed foods like cookies, croutons, and French fries. That can lead to weight loss if you replace those foods with low-calorie options.

THE BAD: A gluten-free diet is not necessarily any healthier than one with gluten. You can still potentially go gluten-free and load up on sugar, gluten-free processed foods, and fatty meats.

THE BOTTOM LINE: There's no evidence that a gluten-free diet provides health benefits if you are not sensitive to gluten. There's really no reason to follow one if you are simply looking for weight loss and health benefits.

Healthy Diet for Weight Control: Back to the "What" and "How Much"

After looking at the above diet patterns, the message remains the same. Eat healthy foods, and keep your portions in check.

As for the "how much," count your calories to be sure you're not taking too much. Aim for 1,000 to 1,200 calories a day while you have the balloon and are under the supervision of your doctor and nutritionist. Bump it up to 1,200 or 1,400 or more calories per day after you get rid of the balloon and if you are losing weight too fast.

Base your diet on vegetables; try to include some at each meal and snack. Reach for vegetables if you're still hungry at a meal or you need an extra snack. These are some additional reminders:

- Include lean proteins at most meals and snacks. Seafood and plant-based proteins, such as beans and soy, may be healthiest, but chicken, eggs, and low-fat dairy are also nutritious.

- Add fruit, whole grains, and starchy vegetables for energy and more nutrients.

- Choose healthy fats, such as nuts, seeds, avocados, flaxseed, and olive oil.

- Limit sugary, fried, and refined foods.

- Drink plenty of water.

Eating right is as simple as it sounds. There are no tricks or gimmicks.

YOUR CHALLENGE

No matter what kind of diet you choose to follow – tradition-al, low-carb, vegetarian, or something else – vegetables are sure to be a part of it. Most vegetables are low in calories and high in nutrients. They're filling, versatile, and easy to prepare. They're even delicious!

Your challenge is to eat more veggies. What does "more" mean? It depends how many you've been eating. Your new goal may be to have a serving every day, or three or even five servings a day. Here are a few ways to squeeze in extra veggies.

- Add them to eggs or a breakfast bowl

- Add them to sandwiches, wraps, burritos, and homemade pizzas

- Add them to sauces and soups

- Use them as side dishes on their own or in salads with potatoes or grains

- Toss them in mixed dishes such as casseroles, chili, stews, and stir fry

- Roast and steam them to serve with any main course

- Have a main course or side salad

- Dip them in Greek yogurt-based dips, peanut butter, or hummus for snacks

THE MEAL PLAN

You can stick to the meal plans you've been following, or you can try a new way of eating. The following vegetarian, vegan, and pescatarian (fish) meal plans have about 1,200 calories just like you've been seeing.

Vegetarian

Meal	Menu
Breakfast	2 whole grain waffles 2 tablespoons almond or peanut butter 1 cup fresh cut or frozen cantaloupe or honeydew melon
Lunch	Cheesy egg salad: • ¼ cup shredded fat-free cheddar cheese • 1 hard-boiled egg • 1 cup diced fresh vegetables of your choice, such as celery, green onion, tomatoes, cucumbers, and mushrooms • ¼ cup Greek yogurt • 1 tablespoon relish (or 1 diced pickle spear) • 1 teaspoon Dijon mustard • ¼ teaspoon paprika Salt and pepper to taste 1 ounce whole-grain pita chips or crackers 1 cup carrot sticks
Dinner	2 portabella pizzas using portabella mushrooms for the crust • Tomato sauce • ½ cup (2 ounces) fat-free mozzarella cheese • Vegetable toppings, such as onions, bell peppers, mushrooms, tomatoes, and olives 1 ounce dark chocolate.

Vegan

Meal	Menu
Breakfast	1 cup unsweetened high-fiber cereal such as shredded wheat ½ cup unsweetened almond milk 2 tablespoons unsweetened shredded coconut 1 banana, sliced.
Lunch	¼ recipe beet and lentil salad with: • 1 cup cooked diced beets • 2 cups cooked lentils (cook in vegetable broth with 1 cup diced carrots for extra flavor) • 1 clove garlic, pressed • ¼ cup red onion, chopped • ½ cup celery, chopped • 1 large tomato, chopped • 2 tablespoons sunflower seeds • 2 tablespoons olive oil • Fresh basil leaves • Lemon juice, parsley, black pepper, and thyme 1 cup fresh fruit salad.
Dinner	"Naked burrito" served on a bed of lettuce with: • ½ cup fat-free vegetarian refried beans • ½ cup cooked brown rice • 1 cup grilled or roasted vegetables such as bell peppers, zucchini, and eggplant • ¼ cup salsa • ¼ cup guacamole 1 sugar-free ice pop

..

Dairy-Free Pescatarian (Fish, No Dairy)

Meal	Menu
Breakfast	Tofu breakfast bowl: • ½ cup tofu • ½ cup garbanzo beans • ½ cup red onion, diced • 2 cups kale • 2 teaspoons olive oil • Salt, garlic powder, cumin, and curry powder to taste ½ grapefruit
Lunch	Salmon salad with 3 ounces cooked salmon on a bed of mixed greens with ½ cup cooked quinoa or barley or brown rice with ½ cup cut fresh fruit such as berries, apples, or pineapple, and 2 tablespoons vinaigrette
Dinner	Shrimp kebabs with: • 4 ounces shrimp • 4 ounces button mushrooms, halved • ½ cup cherry tomatoes or chunks of salad tomatoes • ½ cup red or yellow onions in chunks • ½ cup bell peppers in pieces • Marinade with low-sodium teriyaki sauce and 1 tablespoon olive oil • Brush skewers with marinade and roast or grill ½ acorn squash, roasted.

Chapter 10

Post-Balloon: It's All in Your Hands

CONGRATULATIONS ON MAKING it this far! You've worked with the balloon for months now. You've learned a lot about nutrition, health, and your body, you've developed a lot of healthy habits, and you're well on your way to your weight-loss goals.

Now it is time to get the balloon out of your stomach and to prepare for a future without the balloon. It may seem scary, but you have the tools you need for success.

Getting the Balloon Removed – What to Expect

You may be asked not to eat anything for 24 hours before getting the balloon out. You may also need to avoid drinking any liquids for 12 hours before the removal. The reason is to avoid the risk of aspiration, or choking on food or drink that can make its way to your lungs when you are under sedation.

The procedure takes about 20 minutes under conscious sedation. When you go home, plan to rest. It can take up to three days to fully recover, so avoid strenuous activities. You may feel tired or light-headed.

Stick to clear liquids for the first 24 hours after the system is removed. You can have the same clear liquids as you had when you first got the balloon; for example, water, broth, gelatin, tea, and apple juice. You can also suck on ice chips. Gradually add in more foods as you start to feel up to it.

Staying Motivated

The six-month mark, or the time when you get the balloon out, is a time for celebration. You deserve it! You worked hard for months. You lost weight, cleaned up your eating habits, and improved your health. You should be riding high!

But what will happen when the honeymoon period is over? There may be a time when the weight loss journey isn't as exciting. Without the gastric balloon, you may be less motivated or feel tempted to stray from your healthy intentions. Weight loss may slow or stop, even if you eat right, as you get closer to your goal weight.

You can keep your motivation up by continuing to focus on progress. Weight loss may no longer be as quick and predictable, but you can focus on other measures of progress that can keep you inspired and working hard.

One thing you can do is to set goals for yourself that aren't tied to the scale. You could aim to run a 5k without stopping. You could set the goal of fitting into your dream dress. You could set mini goals linked to the number of pushups, squats, or lunges you can do in a minute.

You can also set challenges for yourself that are linked to behaviors, or process, rather than outcomes. You could challenge yourself to exercise 20 days in the coming month, or eat vegetables for an afternoon snack five days this week. You could pledge to bring your lunch to work four days this week, or cook at least two healthy dishes on the weekend.

Don't forget to reward yourself for your hard work! Stay away from unhealthy food rewards. Instead, find meaning and pleasure in non-food rewards or in healthy food rewards. Consider a spa day or a quick massage, a new outfit for work or for workouts, or something totally unrelated to health, like a movie with a friend. You can also treat yourself to a few downloads so you can beef up your soundtrack for workouts.

Stay away from going off your diet by rewarding yourself with things like big dinners and heavy desserts. Still, it's okay to reward yourself with *healthy* food rewards. For example, you could treat yourself to a pre-made, take-home meal from the supermarket or a family-sized salad with chicken from a local restaurant so you don't have to cook. Or, you could go take a healthy cooking class.

These kinds of rewards acknowledge the hard work you've put in, while also giving you additional motivation to keep moving forward in your healthy ways.

Integrate Your New Habits into Your Life

It's hard enough to work every day for months to eat healthy and exercise. That's what you've been doing for as long as you've had the balloon.

If you're going to keep up these healthy behaviors, though, you need to make them automatic. It's too hard to think consciously every single day about making the right choices. You'll get tired of it sooner or later and likely slip up.

The new habits you've been working so hard to build will stick around longer if you make them part of your life. Build your life so that your healthy behaviors are natural.

You already know to clean out the bad stuff from your kitchen, and to stock it up with good stuff. When you wake up in the morning, you can cook eggs with spinach and turkey bacon rather than with bacon and hash browns. You can pack your whole grain wrap for lunch rather than use an empty fridge as an excuse to hit the drive-through mid-day. You can cook on the weekend so mid-week you can defrost bean soup for dinner rather than order a pizza.

These healthy choices are all the easy ones because you've set up your kitchen properly. You can also set up your life properly to promote health.

- Have enough workout clothes to comfortably get you to the next laundry.

- Get plenty of sleep so it's easier to wake up on time to work out and eat breakfast.

You can also make healthy behaviors fun so that if they went away, you'd miss them. For example:

- Join or start a healthy cooking club to learn new recipes. Bonus: a lot of the members will probably be thrilled to double up as your walking partners!

- Follow a dream such as playing basketball or learning ballet. You'll be motivated to get and stay in shape to do this fun activity.

- Start a monthly "Girls' Night In" where your girlfriends all bring a healthy dish to share and a favorite song to dance to.

- Have a weekly date night or family dinner where your significant other and (if applicable) your children all help plan and cook a healthy meal, which you eat after playing tag, taking a nature walk, or having a dance-off.

- Join a walking club so you make a new set of friends whom you don't get to see unless you actually go walking.

These types of activities give you an incentive to keep up your healthy habits.

Taking Care of Yourself: Beyond Food and Activity

Weight loss and health are about more than diet and exercise. You probably already know that taking care of yourself is a "good" thing to do, even if you don't know why, or what "taking care of yourself" really means. Two of the most important favors you can do for yourself are to get enough sleep and to reduce stress.

Sleep Tight

Sleep is not a luxury. It is a necessity. Don't feel guilty about getting enough sleep each night, and don't cheat yourself out of badly needed shut-eye, even if getting to bed on time takes discipline.

You know sleep makes you feel better, but that's just the beginning. Sleep does all kinds of things for your body. In fact, sleep is another of those secret weight loss tools. Depriving yourself of sleep is a quick way to sabotage your efforts.

When you cut yourself short on sleep, you are setting yourself up for serious hunger. Your stomach produces higher levels of a hormone called ghrelin. Ghrelin tells your brain that you are hungry. When levels are high after a night of little sleep, your brain thinks you are extra hungry, even though you do not really need extra food.

At the same, your levels of the hormone leptin drop when you need more sleep. Leptin is a satiety hormone that helps signal your brain to stop eating. When your levels are low, you do

180

not get as strong of a fullness signal as you should, so you can overeat more easily.

Lack of sleep sabotages weight loss in other ways, too.

- It increases levels of cortisol, which is a stress hormone. Cortisol promotes fat storage, so losing weight is harder.

- It makes you feel more tired, so you are less likely to get in your scheduled workout or move throughout the day. The result is a lower calorie burn.

- It makes high-calorie, sugary foods look more appealing, so you are less likely to turn them down in favor of the healthy foods you should be eating.

- People who are sleep-deprived are more likely to snack late – and not on low-calorie options, either!

Do you need more reasons to get enough sleep? There are many. For example, getting enough sleep is about your overall health and well-being, too. It makes you less anxious and increases productivity. It even improves insulin sensitivity and blood sugar control. That lowers risk for diabetes or helps you manage it if you already have it.

The benefits of sleep and effects of sleep deprivation can start after a single night of inadequate sleep, so take each night seriously! These are some tips for getting enough sleep.[13]

- **Keep a consistent sleep schedule.** Go to bed at the same time each night, and get up at the same in the

---

13 The National Sleep Foundation (NSF) has many resources for improving sleep. The website is at

mornings. Don't skimp on sleep during the week and try to make it up on weekends, or stay up late on weekends only to be hit hard on Monday morning.

- **Be comfortable.** Replace your pillow, mattress, or bedclothes if they are not comfortable.

- **Save your bed for sleeping (and sex).** Do not use it for working, reading, playing on your smartphone, or watching television. Your brain and body should learn that it is time to fall asleep when you go to bed.

- **Sleep in a cool, dark, and quiet room**.

- **Put away the electronics** at least 30 minutes before bed. The glare from the screen signals your brain to wake up.

- **Start a bedtime routine to follow.** Your brain and body will learn that it is time to start shutting down when you begin that familiar routine each night. You can read, listen to music, take a shower, or pack up for tomorrow, for example.

- **Avoid caffeine in the evening** and an oversized dinner.

It can take discipline to get to bed on time when there are so many other things to do in your life, but you got the balloon system to lose weight and get healthy. You owe it to yourself to make those goals a priority in the rest of your life, too.

Manage Stress

Stress is another part of life that can actually affect weight loss. Stress is a normal and healthy reaction because it lets you up your game to handle what life throws at you. Stress becomes a problem when you have too much of it or do not handle it well.

As you probably know first-hand, stress can come from all parts of your life.

- Too much pressure to perform at work, working too much, or worrying about losing your job.

- Relationships at home, with work colleagues, and with friends and more distant family members.

- Worrying about your family members.

Letting stress get the upper hand can harm your health and also get in the way of weight loss. You may already know that stress can raise blood pressure, give you headaches, drain your energy, and interfere with sleep and concentration. Risk for heart disease and diabetes can increase if too much stress continues for too long.

It can also get in the way of weight loss. Just like sleep deprivation, stress affects your hormone levels and your food choices. These are some results of stress:

- Higher levels of stress hormones such as cortisol (remember this metabolism-dropping hormone from lack of sleep?). This hormone also increases appetite.

- Turning to high-calorie comfort foods to calm yourself down

- Increased fat storage, especially around your belly

- Sudden hunger due to the stress hormones digging into your body's stores of carbohydrates as a quick source of energy

You can't avoid all sources stress in your life, but you can prevent stress from harming you. The trick is to remove the ones you can, and to better manage the stress that is unavoidable.

- Don't worry about things you can't control.

- Have one or more go-to people to talk over your minor and major stressors.

- Pinpoint exactly what you're worrying about. Sometimes an undefined worry can cause a lot of stress, but can seem insignificant when you identify exactly what you're worried about.

- Plan ahead so you're not caught scrambling at the last minute.

- Set aside a few minutes to meditate or relax every day.

- Practice relaxation techniques such as deep breathing to turn to when you face a potentially negative situation.

- Eat well and take your vitamins.

Stress is not something to be proud of or fall victim to. It can make you sick and stop weight loss, so do what you can to manage it, even if it takes some effort.

You Are in Good Hands – Yours

You are practically an expert by now. You know everything you need to know about nutrition and healthy foods. You can build a meal plan and prepare healthy meals. You know how to use aids such as food-logging apps.

The balloon may be out, but you're still on the weight loss path. And you have the best possible ally and expert: you. You have the ability to stay on the path you want to be on. You have the ability to help yourself get back on track should you stray. Here are a few thoughts on going forward into your healthy future.

Back to the Basics

It feels bad any time you stray and the number shows up on the scale. You may be disappointed in yourself or feel angry. You might be frustrated if you are not sure what went wrong and what to do about it.

The first step in getting back on track is to realize that you got off track. That's the point at which you realize that the scale isn't lying. For example, you realize that the long plateau or jump in your weight really is a reflection that something is not going right, and it's not just one of those normal fluctuations that happen on a daily basis.

The next step is to forgive yourself, even if it sounds silly or un-necessary. You can move forward much better when you are at peace with yourself. Staying angry with yourself for straying shows that you are not ready to move on. So, forgive and forget.

When you're ready to move forward, you can put yourself back on track by going back to the basics. Think about what you learned when you first got the balloon system. You learned about making the right food choices, cutting back your portions, and eating for hunger without stuffing yourself. You learned how to log your food, eat slowly, and commit to exercise.

Are you as diligent now as you were at the beginning? Or have you let a few things slip? Do you log every bite, chew your food slowly, and eat only after you sit down at the table? Do you snack on vegetables, or slip in some treats that you didn't used to include? Be honest, and you can get back on track.

Back On Track Checklist

This checklist can give you some guidance when you're ready to get back on track but do not know where to start.

- ☐ Log your food so you know for sure how many calories you are getting.
- ☐ Measure your food to make sure your portions are what you think they are. You may need to get your scale and measuring cups and spoons out again, and take smaller portions.
- ☐ Compare the foods you eat to the foods listed in Appendix A and Appendix B. You may need to eat more foods from the Healthy Foods lists and fewer foods from the Not-So-Healthy Foods list.
- ☐ Take note every time you eat about where you are eating. You may need to stop nibbling on the go, and make an effort to eat only sitting down.
- ☐ Track your exercise for a few weeks to check wheth-

er you're getting in as much as you think you are.
You may need to be a little more consistent at the
gym, or get in a few more steps each day.

- ☐ Count the number of ounces of water (or low-calorie liquids) you are drinking each day. It should be
  at least 8 to 12 8-ounce cups, or 64 to 96 ounces,
  per day. You may need to drink a little more.
- ☐ Count the number of hours of sleep you are getting each night. Most adults need 8, and you may
  need even more. Try sleeping without an alarm
  clock. If you sleep past the time you usually set
  your alarm for, you probably need more sleep.
- ☐ Think about the stress in your life. Is it weighing
  on you? You may need to address some stressful
  situations or go back to your stress management
  techniques.
- ☐ Take your time to go through each item on the
  checklist. Don't be afraid. You already know how
  to do each of the things you need to do to lose
  weight, since you learned them and practiced
  them for months while you had the gastric balloon.
  You are sure to see results when you are sure you
  have accomplished each task!

Use Your Health Network

You can do a lot on your own, but healthcare professionals can
certainly help give you information, encouragement, and support. Keep open communication with your healthcare team to
boost your results.

- ■ Your primary care physician (or a specialist if you
  happen to see one more regularly) can encourage
  you during visits and "official" weigh-ins, give you
  blood tests to monitor nutrient levels such as iron

and vitamin D, and check your risk factors such as blood pressure, cholesterol, and blood sugar.

- Your gastric balloon doctor can answer questions about staying on track with weight loss and modifying your diet and lifestyle for long-term changes.

- Your nutritionist can help you design customized meal plans that work for you, give you tips and tricks for making your diet healthier, point out where your diet might be falling short, and give you recipe ideas.

YOUR CHALLENGE

Your challenge this week is to go back to the basics. After six months with the balloon system, you might have slipped a little in your super strict habits. It's possible you're eating a bit of junk food, serving yourself without measuring portion size, or not exercising quite as much as you were.

So, your challenge for this month and any time you feel you may be slipping is to go back to using your basic tracking tools. Spend a week logging everything: from food to weight to fluids to activity and even to sleep. You may find you have a bit of room for improvement – which is great news because fixing those little slip-ups can help you blast through plateaus!

You can come back to this challenge any time you feel you need a little bit of a boost to get back on track. It always works!

THE MEAL PLAN

Your calories will probably increase from the 1,000 to 1,200 you may have been eating when you have the gastric balloon system inside of you. These meal plans provide 1,400 calories. You may need even more calories if you find that you are losing weight too fast, if you add in high amounts of exercise, or if you hit your goal weight. You can always add in more calories by adding healthy snacks and increasing portion sizes, as discussed earlier!

Meal 1

Meal	Menu
Breakfast	1 English muffin ½ cup non-fat cottage cheese 1 medium pear
Lunch	Bean and cheese burrito: ✓ 1 small high-fiber, low-carb tortilla or wrap. ✓ ½ cup fat-free refried beans ✓ ¼ cup fat-free shredded cheddar cheese ✓ 1 cup grilled zucchini 1 cup watermelon 1 ounce whole grain pretzels
Dinner	Spaghetti and meatballs: ✓ ½ cup cooked whole-wheat spaghetti ✓ ½ cup tomato sauce mixed with ½ cup cooked vegetables such as green beans, carrots, or cauliflower ✓ Turkey meatballs with 3 ounces ground turkey, Italian seasoning, 1 egg white, and ¼ cup oats 1 cup steamed broccoli. ½ cup non-fat frozen yogurt. ½ cup strawberries.

Meal 2

Meal	Menu
Breakfast	Quinoa breakfast bowl with: • ½ cup cooked quinoa • 2 eggs, cooked • 1 cup sprouts, such as alfalfa • ¼ avocado • ½ to 1 cup chopped tomato • 3 ounces cooked lean ground turkey, seasoned with Mexican or taco seasoning (optional) • Lime juice (optional)
Lunch	3-4 cups mixed greens or Romaine lettuce mixed with: • 2 tablespoons walnut pieces • ½ cup cooked sweet potato in cubes • ¼ cup parmesan cheese • Vinaigrette with 1 tablespoon olive oil, 1 tablespoon balsamic vinegar, and dried oregano and rosemary 1 cup strawberries or other fruit
Dinner	Black bean chicken stir fry: • 4 ounces skinless chicken breast, cut in pieces • ½ cup mung bean sprouts • ½ cup broccoli • ½ cup mushrooms • 2 tablespoons black bean sauce • 2 teaspoons sesame oil • 1 tablespoon rice wine vinegar Marinated pepper salad (make the night before) • 1 cup cut bell peppers (such as green, red, or yellow) • 1 diced green onion. • 1 tablespoon rice wine or red wine vinegar • 2 teaspoons capers • 2 teaspoons olive oil • 1 packet calorie-free sugar substitute • Salt and pepper to taste

Appendices

Appendix A: Healthy Food Lists

Diet Foundation

Non-starchy vegetables

- Almost all vegetables: artichokes, carrots, peppers, eggplant, tomatoes, spinach, cabbage, broccoli, beets, zucchini, mushrooms...and so on!

- Salad greens: lettuce, spinach, and mixed greens

- "Snacking" vegetables, such as cucumbers, celery, baby carrots, and cherry tomatoes

- Canned tomatoes

- Frozen vegetables

- Be careful of: frozen and canned vegetables with added sugar and/or salt

Legumes

- Beans: canned low-sodium and dried garbanzo, kidney, black, navy, pinto, and others

- Peas: dried split peas, yellow peas, and black-eyed peas

- Lentils: dried lentils

- Canned low-sodium bean, lentil, and pea soup

Lean Proteins

- Eggs, egg whites, and liquid egg whites

- Skinless chicken and turkey

- Lean ground turkey and soy crumble.

- Veggie burgers

- Fish and shellfish

- Canned seafood and seafood in pouches, such as sardines, tuna, clams, oysters, mackerel, and salmon

- Tofu

- Be careful of: processed meats such as ham, other deli meats, and sausage (high-sodium, nitrates)

Starches: Healthy Grains and Starchy Vegetables

- Plain and no sugar added oatmeal

- Other whole grain hot cereals, such as ancient grains and whole grain farina

- Whole grain cold breakfast cereal, such as Fiber One, shredded wheat, and All-Bran

- Bulgur, barley, quinoa, whole wheat couscous, and other whole grains

- Whole grain bread and pasta

- Brown rice

- Whole grain pretzels and crackers

- Plain popcorn

- Potatoes, sweet potatoes, winter squash such as kabocha, butternut, and acorn, peas, and corn

- Be careful of: sweetened hot and cold cereals (high-calorie and high-sugar); fried potatoes such as French fries and hash browns (high-calorie and high-fat)

Fruit

- Fresh fruit

- Frozen fruit with no sugar added

- Be careful of: dried fruit (high in sugar); fruit juice (high in sugar, low in fiber); frozen and canned fruit with added sugar

Healthy Fats

- Avocados

- Nuts, such as almonds, cashews, walnuts, and pecans, and nut butters

- Peanuts and peanut butter

- Seeds, such as pumpkin, flax, and sunflower

- Olive oil

- Other vegetable oils such as canola, flaxseed, and sesame

- Be careful of: too-big serving sizes (high-calorie); processed foods such as peanut butter (includes un-healthy hydrogenated fats)

Better-Choice Condiments

- Vinegar, such as balsamic, white wine, red wine, and rice wine

- Vinaigrette and light salad dressing

- Salsa

- Mustard (not honey mustard): yellow, deli, spicy brown, Dijon

- Hot sauce, such as sriracha, Louisiana hot sauce, or harissa

- Cocktail, steak, and Worcestershire sauce

- Soy sauce (choose low-sodium)

- Horseradish

- Teriyaki sauce (watch the portion size because it can be high-sugar)

- Ketchup (watch the portion size because it can be high-sugar)

- Fresh and dried herbs and spices

- Low-sodium seasoning and spice mixes

- Reduced-calorie salad dressings, salad spritzers

Appendix B: List of Not So Healthy Foods

Food	Reason and Alternative	
Processed meats, such as bacon, salami, sausage, pepperoni, and ham	They're high-sodium and often high-fat; they also usually have nitrates, which cause cancer.	Low-fat alternatives, such as all-natural turkey bacon and vegetarian sausage; unprocessed meats, such as chicken breast; low-sodium and all-natural, nitrate-free ham and deli turkey.
Fatty meats, such as bacon, sausage, ribs, fatty steaks, and regular ground beef.	They're high in calories and unhealthy saturated fat.	Meats without visible fat; skinless chicken or turkey; meatless substitutes such as veggie burgers or soy bacon.
Butter and lard	They're high in unhealthy saturated fat.	Cooking spray or olive or another plant-based oil for cooking; try avocado or hummus as a spread on sandwiches; use peanut butter on toast; substitute non-fat sour cream or pumpkin puree in baked goods.
Desserts, such as cake, pie, cookies, and ice cream	They're usually high in calories, sugars, and unhealthy fats.	Fresh fruit as an everyday dessert or snack; smaller portions for an occasional treat; frozen Greek yogurt as an ice cream swap.
Fried foods, such as onion rings, fried chicken, fried shrimp, French fries, and doughnuts.	They're high in calories because of the fat from frying, and they can have unhealthy trans fats.	Baked alternatives, such as baked zucchini fries instead zucchini sticks, baked "fried" chicken instead of regular, and grilled shrimp instead of fried.

Food	Reason and Alternative	
Unhealthy potatoes, such as French fries, mashed potatoes, and potato chips	They're high in carbs and calories and high in fat.	Non-fried, potato-free options, such as baked sweet potato fries instead of French fries, pureed cauliflower instead of mashed potatoes, and baked kale chips instead of potato chips. Small baked potatoes with broccoli and cheese are another choice.
Refined snack foods, such as chips, white crackers, and pretzels	They're usually high in calories, sodium, and refined carbs.	Whole grain options, such as air popped popcorn, whole wheat pretzels, and brown rice cakes. Nuts are also a crunchy snack option – just watch portion sizes. You can also crunch zucchini and radish chips, dried seaweed snacks, roasted soybeans and garbanzo beans, and raw vegetables.
Refined grains, such as white bread, pasta, and rice, and refined cereals	They're high-glycemic, which means they spike your blood sugar. They're also high in calories and low in fiber.	Whole grain options, such as whole wheat bread and pasta and brown rice, and fortified whole grain cereals.
Jams, jellies, preserves, honey, and maple syrup	They're high in sugar and calories and low in nutrients.	Fresh fruit for sandwiches and pancake toppings; low-sugar jam and syrup; applesauce and reduced-calorie sweeteners for baking.
Sugar-sweetened otherwise healthy foods, such as yogurt, cereal, and frozen and canned fruit	They have extra calories and sugar, often in the form of corn syrup.	Unsweetened versions, such as plain or no sugar added yogurt, unsweetened whole grain cereal, and frozen fruit with no added sugar.

Food	Reason and Alternative	
Sugar-sweetened beverages, like sodas, sports drinks, fruit drinks, and sweetened coffee and tea	They're high in sugar and calories, and low in nutrients.	Calorie-free or low-calorie beverages such as water, flavored water, and decaffeinated unsweetened tea and coffee.

Appendix C: Healthy Snack Lists

Each meal plan shows three meals per day that total approximately 1,000 to 1,200 calories. If you need more calories than that, you can add in healthy snacks. These are some healthy snacks to try at the 100, 150, and 200-calorie levels.

100 or Fewer Calories

- 2 ounces all-natural turkey spread with ½ cup "Broccomole" made with pureed broccoli, garlic, lemon or lime juice, and cilantro

- 1 low-fat string cheese stick (mozzarella cheese) and 1 tangerine

- ½ whole grain English muffin spread with 2 tablespoons non-fat cream cheese with lettuce and tomato slices

- 2 ounces (1/4 cup) tuna mixed with 2 tablespoons non-fat Greek yogurt spread on celery sticks

About 150 Calories

- 1 cup watermelon tossed with 1 ounce feta cheese tossed (optional) with basil and black pepper

- ½ cup non-fat cottage cheese with 1 cup cut cantaloupe

- 1 ounce pistachio or cashew nuts

- 2 hard-boiled eggs

- 2 ounces (1/4 cup) guacamole plus 1 cup cauliflower florets

- ½ cup fat-free refried beans with 1 ounce fat-free cheese melted on top

- ¼ cup roasted edamame (green soybeans)

- Chicken salad with ½ cup diced chicken, ¼ cup plain Greek yogurt, pepper, Dijon mustard, and diced pickle served on a bed of lettuce

- ½ cup bran flakes, ½ cup unsweetened almond milk, and ½ sliced banana

200 or More Calories

- 2 brown rice cakes with 1 tablespoon peanut or almond butter

- 1 diced medium apple with ½ ounce walnuts and ½ cup grapes

- 1 container fat-free plain or no sugar added Greek yogurt plus 1 ounce whole grain cereal or oats

- 1 cup whole grain salad made with ½ cup cooked whole grain (such as quinoa, barley, or brown rice) with ½ cup diced vegetables such as cucumber, red pepper, onion, and sweet corn, 2 teaspoons olive oil, and vinegar, pepper, and low-calorie sweetener

- Pizza burrito with 1 small high-fiber tortilla or wrap spread with tomato sauce and filled with ¼ cup shredded mozzarella cheese plus mushrooms, bell peppers, and (optional) anchovies

About the Authors

Alex Brecher

The founder and CEO of BariatricPal, the world's largest online social network dedicated to the weight loss surgery community, Alex Brecher became committed to fighting obesity with weight loss surgery after his own successful lap-band surgery. It helped him to lose over 100 pounds and keep it off for over 14 years. Brecher's years of experience in web design, forum hosting, technology, and management enabled him to establish BariatricPal and guide its development. Brecher has served as a consultant for numerous bariatrics companies, and he supports many professional organizations for weight loss surgery, including the American Society for Bariatric and Metabolic Surgery (ASMBS), International Federation for the Surgery of Obesity and Metabolic Disorders (IFSO), and the Association for the Study of Obesity (ASO). Brecher is a native New Yorker who loves spending time with his three children and staying fit by working out at the gym and running. Brecher and Stein have co-authored four previous books on weight loss surgery.

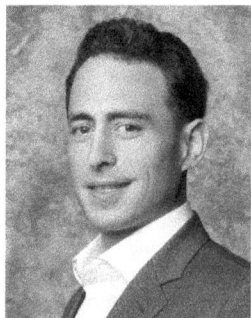

Natalie Stein

Natalie Stein is a writer who specializes in nutrition and weight loss. For years, she has worked with co-author Alex Brecher to maintain the content on BariatricPal. Stein received graduate degrees in nutrition and public health, and teaches graduate courses in public health nutrition at a major university. In addition to co-authoring three books on weight loss surgery with Brecher, Stein has a college textbook on public health nutrition to her credit. Stein is based in Los Angeles. She enjoys talking to friends and family and spending time at the gym, and she is an avid runner who has completed six marathons.

www.ingramcontent.com/pod-product-compliance
Lightning Source LLC
Chambersburg PA
CBHW070804280326
41934CB00012B/3046